"Rachel excels at mak   ng
through medical termin\u0001\u0001\u0001\u0001 ....   -ler
first book is THE guidebook to living with hypothyroidism; and
this follow-up, with husband Adam, picks up right where Be Your
Own Thyroid Advocate left off. How do we approach our loved
ones and teach them not only to assist in advocating for us, but
also to understand our symptoms? Here, Rachel and Adam
provide an insightful, very human map of survival - and remind
us that we are, as ever, never alone."
— Lauren Freedman, Host & Founder of Uninvisible Pod

"Gask's genuine testimony is paired with inspiring words that
are sure to provide motivation and perspective that can help
thyroid patients and their partners make it through the most
challenging of times."
— The National Academy of Hypothyroidism

"For those of us with hypothyroidism, living and thriving
requires far more than just taking a daily pill and monitoring labs.
The real magic of Rachel and Adam's book is that it addresses
each and every aspect of this challenging condition through a dual
lens. It's not only the lives of the diagnosed, but the lives of our
loved ones which are wholly affected. Couples affected by
hypothyroidism should read this book as an insurance policy
against break-up, divorce, and a lot of unnecessary suffering."
— Ginny Mahar, ThyroidRefresh

"You, Me and Hypothyroidism can help bridge barriers to communication and help you support those in your life who struggle with hypothyroidism. I ultimately hope everyone hears about and reads this essential book to greatly improve the quality of life for all those who struggle with hypothyroidism!"
– Zana Carver, Thyroid Code

"Rachel and her partner, Adam, write an inspiring and powerful piece about the reality of loving someone with Hypothyroidism. Their book eloquently reveals a perspective we often overlook, and provides our loved ones with the chance to better understand what we, as Hypothyroid patients, deal with and how to love us through those struggles. You, Me and Hypothyroidism truly embodies the reality of loving someone in sickness and in health. It is a must-read if you know, love and care for someone with Hypothyroidism."
– Victoria, thebutterflyeffectblog.org

Also by The Author

Be Your Own Thyroid Advocate: When You're Sick and Tired of Being Sick and Tired

Covering all the thyroid basics those with hypothyroidism need to know, thyroid patient Rachel Hill wrote *Be Your Own Thyroid Advocate: When You're Sick and Tired of Being Sick and Tired* for those who are relatively new to learning about their thyroid health.

Included in the book:

- A recounting of Rachel's personal journey back to good health with hypothyroidism and Hashimoto's
- The most important information Rachel has learnt along the way so that other thyroid patients can reclaim their health too
- Chapters on thyroid medication, blood tests, supplements, mental health and the other pieces of the puzzle people with hypothyroidism may not have thought about
- A chapter speaking to the friends and family of those with hypothyroidism, including how they can support the thyroid patient in their life
- Motivational and uplifting passages to support thyroid patients in their own journey
- Chapters on dealing with the diagnosis of hypothyroidism and support for remaining in employment
- Thyroid health resources (websites, books and a list of awareness events)

You, Me and Hypothyroidism

When Someone You Love Has Hypothyroidism

Understanding Hypothyroidism and How Your Relationship Can Still Thrive

RACHEL HILL AKA THE INVISIBLE HYPOTHYROIDISM
AND
ADAM GASK

Copies are available at special rates for bulk orders.
Contact rachel@theinvisiblehypothyroidism.com for more information.

Up to date contact information can be found at:
www.theinvisiblehypothyroidism.com

First Edition.

ISBN: 978-1-91609-031-6

Dedications

Dedication from Rachel

To my wonderful friends and family who have not only supported me through my diagnoses and the many trials and tribulations with my health, but also sought to understand what it is that I and so many others with thyroid problems experience. We appreciate attempts to understand and help us more than you'll ever know. So thank you.

Dedication from Adam

To Rachel, my best friend, for never giving up. To my mum, dad and auntie who have always been so patient and who support Rachel and I in so many ways. To all the spouses, friends and family supporting and lifting up those with hypothyroidism. You all make a difference, thank you.

Acknowledgements

Thank you to the thyroid community who gave us many suggestions for what to include in this book. We hope to have delivered a useful tool that will help more relationships to thrive despite that third wheel: thyroid disease.

The thyroid patients around the world who very kindly read an early copy of this book and provided us with feedback on content. You helped to ensure we delivered what people were wanting in this book.

Ahmad Shoma, who created the illustration on the cover of this book.

Most importantly, this book or any of The Invisible Hypothyroidism's work would not have been possible without all the thyroid patients worldwide who follow and support The Invisible Hypothyroidism's message. Many of them requested this book and we're pleased to say it's finally here!

Disclaimer

This book is compiled to provide information and education on health. It contains information that is intended to help the reader become a better-informed consumer of healthcare. Its publication is not intended to replace the relationship with your or your loved one's doctor or any other medical professional and their guidance. Neither the publisher, authors, or anyone involved with making this book, mentioned or quoted in the book, takes responsibility for any consequences of any treatment, actions or application of any method by any person reading or following the information contained in this book. You are responsible for your actions relating to your own health and relationships. The authors of this book are not medically trained or trained in counselling or relationship management.

It is recommended that any consumer of this material consult with their physician regarding any drugs, supplements, diet changes or other treatments and therapies that may be beneficial to them. You may also wish to seek relationship counselling. This book is not intended as a substitute for the medical advice of a doctor, or guidance of a relationship or otherwise counsellor or therapist. Any readers should regularly consult a physician in matters relating to their health.

Every effort has been made to ensure that this book is as complete and accurate as possible, however, there may be mistakes, both typographical and in content. This book contains information that should be assumed current only up to the printing date. This book should only be used as a guide and not to replace your relationship with your doctor or anyone else involved in your physical or mental health and well-being.

About the Authors

Rachel Hill, creator of The Invisible Hypothyroidism and nominee of eight 2019 WEGO Health Awards, lives in England with her husband Adam. Although she took his surname legally, she keeps her maiden name professionally.

She is a highly ranked and award-winning thyroid patient advocate, appearing in top thyroid resource lists, as a valued contributor to the thyroid patient community. As well as a passionate thyroid advocate, Rachel enjoys satisfying her wanderlust trait, reading, finding new music and of course: eating.

To keep up to date on thyroid news, information and Rachel's personal journey, please visit her website at TheInvisibleHypothyroidism.com, where you will find she's poured countless hours into providing as much information for thyroid patients as possible.

"I want to inspire and reassure people. I want to give those who really need it, hope. I want to reach someone and have them think 'because of you, I didn't give up.' That's what drives me."

* * *

Adam Gask is a Software Engineer, Business Owner and long-time partner of Rachel. He is often found tinkering over a computer, watching his beloved Leicester City FC or providing "IT Support" for his nearest and dearest.

Contents

Preface

"How wonderful it is to have someone who cares for you so deeply that they wish to understand your plight?" - Rachel Hill, *The Invisible Hypothyroidism*

"loved one"
noun
  1. **a person who is a member of one's family or a close friend. A cherished relationship.**

750 million people around the world have thyroid disease and you know at least one of them. In fact, you probably know *multiple* without even realising.

Thyroid disease isn't spoken about often enough and many people living with it keep it to themselves; worried that others simply won't understand, or may even judge or ridicule them.

This is where *you*, the friend, family member, spouse, partner, work colleague or as we refer to anyone who knows someone with hypothyroidism in this book: **the loved one**, comes in. The fact that you've picked up this book is hugely appreciated. It means a lot that you wish to understand, help and support the thyroid patient in your life.

The aim of writing this book was to provide loved ones with guidance on supporting the thyroid patient in their life but also reassurance that their experiences are valid too. And that's why we, a married couple consisting of a hypothyroid wife and a husband who has supported her, have written this book together.

Providing the experiences as a thyroid patient sharing what I know you can do to support them, I, Rachel, hope to provide you, the loved one, with guidance on supporting the hypothyroid person in your life.

Providing the point of view as an experienced partner of a thyroid patient, Adam gives you someone to relate to as he shares what he has learnt whilst being in a relationship with someone that has hypothyroidism. He validates the struggles of those supporting someone with hypothyroidism and reassures you that you're not alone if you're feeling lost too.

If you're unsure about *how* to help, what you 'should' know or perhaps 'should be doing', he'll provide reassurance that hasn't been given elsewhere at the time of writing this book. In fact, we're astounded, as I often mention in my thyroid advocacy work, that support for those supporting thyroid patients isn't discussed by anyone else. It's completely glossed over, as if thyroid patients should expect their loved ones to 'just know' what to do.

It may be that the thyroid patient in your life has asked you to read this book and for doing so, we say *thank you*. That alone demonstrates your support for helping them figure all of this 'learning to live with chronic illness' stuff out.

Adam knows all too well how lonely and difficult it can be for loved ones to deal with a chronic illness diagnosis too. Adam recounts that he didn't know where to turn to for support in dealing with an ill partner and that turning to his friends didn't come naturally, as he evolved into a 'carer' type role following my decline in health due to thyroid disease. He couldn't find any guidance or support for this change to his life, which made it isolating. We hope this book will provide one such resource.

My first book, *Be Your Own Thyroid Advocate: When You're Sick and Tired of Being Sick and Tired* was written for those living with hypothyroidism, as I recounted my journey and a lot of the things I did to get my health back and thrive with thyroid disease. But this book is for the thyroid patient's nearest and dearest. Whereas *Be Your Own Thyroid Advocate* was a self-help book to aid thyroid patients towards a better quality of life, *You, Me and Hypothyroidism* is, in the same way, here to help those supporting someone with hypothyroidism to also thrive, by learning how to reinforce and maintain a strong relationship despite the challenges that thyroid disease can bring.

I'm not exaggerating when I say that I often hear from thyroid patients whose marriage has broken down due to the strains of hypothyroidism. Who have miscarried pregnancies or cannot conceive children due to complications of hypothyroidism. Who have lost friends and fell out with family due to the effects of hypothyroidism on their social lives, ability to work, run a household or even in tolerating stress that others can seemingly tolerate so much easier.

Yes, hypothyroidism can be a real test on relationships, whether they're romantic, familial, professional relationships or friendships.

So, we both hope this book shines more light on hypothyroidism and creates even more room to discuss the difficulties, struggles and issues surrounding the condition. We hope it can *save* relationships, marriages, friendships and more from being negatively affected by a condition that ironically isn't even well-recognised by the general public.

You, Me and Hypothyroidism focuses on strengthening relationships via awareness and validation, which is an important part of adjusting to any lifelong condition. For all involved and affected.

They often say that the strongest relationships are those that have endured hardships and challenges but come out of it stronger and more resilient. Hypothyroidism can be a challenge. A real challenge. But you *can* come out of it with a reinforced relationship and even deeper connection to the person you love, who just so happens to also be a thyroid patient.

Rachel Hill, The Invisible Hypothyroidism

Rachel's Introduction

"I am spending the rest of my life making other people feel less lost." - Rachel Hill, The Invisible Hypothyroidism

I already promote that each thyroid patient should embrace being their own healthcare advocate, but I must also promote that we seek to build a strong support network around us, too.

The standard thyroid medication and treatment for hypothyroidism is a hormone replacement drug, called thyroxine, which many thyroid patients respond absolutely fine to and find that they can live life pretty much as they did before they developed hypothyroidism. But as with everything, there are some who have that experience and then some who do not.

There are thyroid patients around the world who take their medication and still feel hugely unwell. Every aspect of their lives affected in some way or another, from social life to work life and even love life. For these people, adapting and adjusting can include a whole mix of emotions. Whilst they try to figure out how to get back to good health, just as I eventually did and have recounted through my blog and in my first book, a strong support network will be required. And due to life with thyroid disease often being quite an up and down affair, maintaining an open discussion and understanding of what you're both experiencing will be crucial.

Adam and I met at fifteen years old and started dating at sixteen. Now in our mid-twenties, we've spent ten years together and in those ten years, have experienced a lot more than your average couple of our age. One thing we experienced was my decline in health and being diagnosed with a chronic illness at just twenty-one years old.

It hasn't been an easy adjustment and we're still learning as we *both* go along on this eventful thyroid journey. However, after getting through the darkest and most difficult of times with this disease, we've already got a lot to share with other people in similar relationships.

If you've ever started a new hobby, workout routine or commitment, you probably know how much help having the support of another person can be. You also probably know how easy it is to fall off the wagon when starting out but with someone there to help you keep your goals in sight and work towards, there's a better chance of accomplishing them. And this is where you can be immensely useful in the recovery of the person you know with hypothyroidism.

You may ask what experience I have to write this book. I started out my work as a thyroid patient advocate by blogging about my own experiences and this soon evolved into a lot more. Writing for various other websites, doing interviews and podcasts, running online support groups and working with The BBC, The National Academy of Hypothyroidism, ThyroidChange and more, I also contributed to a thyroid cookbook in 2018 before releasing *Be Your Own Thyroid Advocate.*

I have experience as a thyroid patient and as an advocate for raising awareness of hypothyroidism. In 2019 I was also nominated for eight WEGO Health Awards.

But I can't claim to say I have experience as someone who lives with, works with, is related to or friends with someone who has hypothyroidism. And that's why I write this book with Adam, my now husband, to ensure we get the balance right.

Rachel Hill, The Invisible Hypothyroidism

Adam's Introduction

"Life is like riding a bicycle. To keep your balance, you must keep moving." - Albert Einstein

Firstly, well done for picking up this book. You've done something that most people in your situation simply don't do.

In this book, I hope to give you an insight into the things that have helped me through Rachel's hypothyroidism journey. I'll talk about understanding the thyroid patient in your life's energy levels, how different days can mean different things, and how by learning some key things, both of you can thrive. Most importantly, I want to ensure that you know and understand that whilst supporting your loved one is incredibly important, it is also important to look after yourself. By ensuring that you're setup with the knowledge and information you need, things can and will get easier. However, unless you have the ability to manage your own mental health and well-being, trying to support someone with a chronic illness can be an incredible strain.

I aim for my contributions to this book to be quite conversational, and be the sort of advice that you can interpret for your own situation, and hopefully feel a little less alone in this journey.

You will find that the book is split into four parts, with Part One applicable to anyone who knows someone with hypothyroidism as it covers a lot of the basics, Part Two suitable for romantic relationships as it looks at things like libido, fertility, pregnancy etc. Part Three for anyone who lives with a thyroid patient as well as friends and family, as it discusses effects on social life, work life and dietary changes, and Part Four is for supporting all loved ones. You will get the most out of this book by reading it all, but you may wish to skip straight to the bits that apply to you first.

Passages written by myself will appear in this font and although much of my experience is with a female partner with hypothyroidism and Hashimoto's, we have kept in mind that anyone can have thyroid disease, so have made a point to not only focus on female thyroid patients and romantic relationships.

Adam Gask

Part One: Everyone is Welcome

Information for anyone and everyone who knows someone with hypothyroidism.

Chapter 1: An Open Letter

"No two people are exactly the same, which means that no two people will heal exactly the same." - Rachel Hill, The Invisible Hypothyroidism

As a thyroid patient advocate, one of my most popular articles has been the open letter I wrote to those who know someone with hypothyroidism.

This open letter was written with the aim of giving those who know someone with hypothyroidism a better understanding of what it is we go through as patients and how they can help us.

It felt like the perfect way to begin this book and introduce you to *You, Me and Hypothyroidism: When Someone You Love Has Hypothyroidism.*

An Open Letter to Those Who Know Someone with Hypothyroidism

Hello friend, family member, work colleague or doctor of someone who lives with an underactive thyroid or hypothyroidism. You know someone very strong, battling an often-difficult disease.

If you're not a medical professional, you're probably wondering what exactly an underactive thyroid or hypothyroidism is, or how it affects someone who lives with it, so I'll do my best to explain it as simply as possible.

You've likely already heard some things about it, for example that it is an excuse people use for being overweight. But this is far from what it really does to someone. In reality, hypothyroidism does so much more to its host. It hurts when we see people use the term "thyroid problem" as code to describe someone who is overweight. It also belittles the condition. It's so much worse than just weight gain, although this is still a legitimate symptom.

The thyroid gland is located in the neck and its hormones are required for every cell and function of the body. An underactive thyroid means just that; it's under active. It's slow and sluggish and not performing properly, meaning a slow metabolism that causes weight gain and very little energy, as well as lots of other symptoms. The same goes for those who are hypothyroid through having no thyroid gland at all.

For the thyroid gland to function properly, we need the right amount of thyroid hormones in our bodies. If we don't have these, it affects our energy levels and lots of other things, especially things you probably don't even think about. For example, sleep cycles, body temperature, alertness, thinking clearly, appetite and fertility, to name just a few.

Hypothyroidism is most commonly caused by an autoimmune disease, such as Hashimoto's Thyroiditis or Graves' Disease. Sometimes it is caused by having treatment for hyperthyroidism (an overactive thyroid) or having had treatment for thyroid cancer. The treatment often used for these, radioactive iodine treatment or a thyroidectomy, can result in the patient becoming hypothyroid. So, any of these could have caused the person you know to have the condition.

You may even know another person with hypothyroidism, who takes medication for it and is seemingly OK, but this isn't the same for all thyroid patients. Actually, a lot of thyroid patients find it's not easily treated and controlled. The other person you know may not have told you the full extent of how it affects them, either.

Hypothyroidism can cause mental health conditions like depression and anxiety, as well as physical symptoms like loss of hair, brain fog, aches and pains throughout the body, constipation, an increase or decrease in blood pressure and even scary heart palpitations and loss of appetite, to name just a few.

You can imagine that a lack of sleep, or needing to sleep lots but actually not feeling any better when we do, may make the simplest of everyday tasks difficult or impossible for a thyroid patient.

The best way I can describe hypothyroidism symptoms is by comparing it to the flu. The fatigue and aches are very similar. You know how frustrated, fed-up and useless you feel when you're ill and have things to do? That's how it can be to have hypothyroidism. Except we have no choice but to work, run a family, house, maintain a social life (or at least try to) and try to maintain a positive attitude towards life.

Combine it with all of these symptoms here:

- Constipation
- Depression
- Slow movements, speech and thoughts
- Itchy and/or sore scalp
- Muscle cramps
- Dry and tight feeling skin
- Brittle hair and nails
- Pain, numbness and a tingling sensation
- Irregular periods or heavy periods
- Brain fog/confusion/memory problems
- Migraines
- Hoarse voice
- A puffy-looking face
- Thinned or partly missing eyebrows
- Poor stamina
- Long recovery period after any activity
- Arms feeling like dead weights after activity
- Inability to exercise, or withstand certain exercises
- Tendency to be overly emotional
- Inability to tolerate cold – cold hands and feet
- Poor circulation
- High or rising cholesterol
- Acid reflux
- Swollen legs that impede walking

- Difficulty standing on feet
- Joint stiffness and pain
- Fertility issues

and you get the picture of what it's like.

So, you can imagine that sometimes, thyroid patients living with these have to cancel plans last minute, through no fault of their own. When they have plans to do something, they tend to look forward to it, as it can take their mind off their health condition or make them feel like they're taking back some control. So, if they then have to cancel on you due to hypothyroid symptoms and struggles, you can imagine how devastated they likely feel. The next time you think they might be making up excuses, being lazy or being a cop-out, please realise that when this is their life, they have no real control and they are not to blame.

We didn't *choose* to have thyroid disease.

Thyroid patients are often not easily understood by those around them. We're made to feel like this condition isn't a big thing to live with as it is often not taken seriously. Most people think it's an easily treated condition, when in reality, it is none of those things for many patients. We're not hypochondriacs, it really does cause lots of symptoms.

Yes, for some thyroid patients they do OK on standard thyroid medication but for many, they still struggle.

Even some of our friends, family and work colleagues (this could be you) overlook how serious it is, and how detrimental it can be to our lives. Even some doctors look at it like this. Not all, but a lot. A lot more than we should have to experience when fighting to regain some quality of life.

Many patients struggle to actually get diagnosed for years, with doctors brushing it off as depression, chronic fatigue syndrome or fibromyalgia, among other things. Doctors regularly misdiagnose hypothyroidism. Even when we are diagnosed and started on medication, we often find it takes some time to feel better, or that doctors will not consider another type of medication if the first one they try doesn't work for us. A lot of us even have to turn to going private for our healthcare or sourcing the medication ourselves. So don't assume that your friend, family member or work colleague is 'OK now they've got medication for it'. Instead, please ask us.

Can you imagine how lonely we feel sometimes? Alone in our struggles and feeling like no one understands?

What we would like from you is to be the person who understands what we're going through, and that even though it's not a well-recognised disease, it is a real, difficult, life-changing condition. It often destroys, changes and alters lives forever.

The best thing you can do is to be there for your friend, family member or work colleague who has this disease; all we need you to do is listen, and learn about the struggles and challenges we face. We don't expect you to know everything, but to be understanding and sympathetic when we are struggling. You could help the thyroid patient in your life do as much as possible to improve their health, be it encourage them to seek out a doctor who will listen, or do research with them to learn more about how they can help themselves feel better.

When they read a new book, read it with them. Thyroid brain fog can make us forget a lot of what we read! Encourage them to pick up new thyroid books. Be the person who helps them to find time for rest, self-care and time to enjoy what they love doing most. It might be helpful for you to read about other patients' experiences, too. Ask us if we need help with anything and ask us how we've been feeling. It's good to know someone cares.

If you live with a thyroid patient, don't expect too much from them in daily life. I'm not saying that all thyroid patients are incapable of doing anything, far from it actually, but rather that you shouldn't expect them to do as much as they used to. Instead, let them rediscover their limits and stamina.

You may have to take up more of the housework and take initiative on things that they used to be in charge of in order to help. Tell them when they've done enough for the day and encourage them to rest. Bring them drinks, run them a bath, or simply ask if they need help getting up the stairs or putting their shoes on. Go with them to doctor appointments and help them get the right treatment for them. Encourage them to find online support groups and networks to meet others also living with the disease. Often, experience and advice can be shared among patients, which is invaluable to helping make the condition that little bit easier to live with.

Something as simple as reading this letter, means the world to us. It means a lot that you want to understand our situation and help us, or at least be someone we can talk and rant to, and rely on to listen to us when we're having a hard day.

* * *

Chapter 2: Understanding Hypothyroidism

"There is nothing in nature that blooms every day, all year long. So we won't either." - Rachel Hill, The Invisible Hypothyroidism

What on Earth is hypothyroidism anyway? That's something I suspect many of you first thought when hearing about the disease for the first time. It is clearly important to cover what hypothyroidism is in a book about hypothyroidism, but if you already know a lot of this then A) I'm really impressed and B) Sorry!

Hypothyroidism can go by a few different names. You may have heard of:

- An Underactive Thyroid
- Low Thyroid
- Thyroid Disease
- Thyroid Disorder
- Thyroid Condition
- Thyroid Problem
- Autoimmune Hypothyroidism

Which can all be different names for hypothyroidism, though not every one of them applies to every person with hypothyroidism. Which one should you be using for the person you know?

The Difference in Names

An Underactive Thyroid

The term 'underactive thyroid' is perhaps the most well-recognised term among the general public. It is used when the thyroid gland isn't producing as much thyroid hormone as it should be, therefore being 'under active', and resulting in a long list of symptoms.

Thyroid hormone is needed for every process, every cell and every function in the body. An underactive thyroid is most often caused (90% of the time)[1] by the autoimmune disease Hashimoto's. However, if someone doesn't have a thyroid gland, i.e. are born without a thyroid, have had it removed due to thyroid cancer or have had it ablated (meaning all function destroyed) then the term an "underactive thyroid" isn't used for them as they don't have a working thyroid gland at all, let alone one that is underactive.

So, the term 'underactive thyroid' is suitable for your loved one if:

- They have a thyroid gland that isn't producing enough thyroid hormone, whether it is due to having the autoimmune disease Hashimoto's or not
- They have subclinical/borderline hypothyroidism

Hypothyroidism

Usually the most appropriate term for most kinds of conditions resulting from inadequate levels of thyroid hormone, 'hypothyroidism' means to have low thyroid hormone levels, and this can be from having no thyroid gland at all, only part of one, or having a thyroid that doesn't work properly (from Hashimoto's or other causes).

So, the term 'hypothyroidism' is suitable for your loved one if:

- They have a thyroid gland that isn't producing enough thyroid hormone, whether it is due to the autoimmune disease Hashimoto's or something else
- They do not have a thyroid gland
- They have a thyroid gland that has lost all function (i.e. ablated)
- They have part of a full thyroid gland that isn't producing enough thyroid hormone
- They have subclinical/borderline hypothyroidism
- They have congenital hypothyroidism (hypothyroidism present from birth)

Low Thyroid

'Low thyroid', most often used by doctors and in medical books, is the same as 'hypothyroidism'. It means to have low thyroid hormone levels. See 'hypothyroidism' above.

Thyroid Disease, Thyroid Disorder, Thyroid Condition, Thyroid Problem

These tend to be used when the structure or function of the thyroid gland is affected in some way. Therefore, they can cover anything being abnormal with the thyroid gland.

So, these terms are suitable for your loved one if:

- They have a thyroid gland that isn't producing enough thyroid hormone, whether it is due to autoimmune disease Hashimoto's or something else
- They have a thyroid gland that is producing too much thyroid hormone, whether it is due to autoimmune disease Graves' or something else
- They have thyroid cancer
- They do not have a thyroid gland
- They have part of a full thyroid gland that isn't producing enough thyroid hormone
- They have a thyroid gland that has lost all function (i.e. ablated)
- They have subacute thyroiditis or other short-term thyroid disorder
- They have subclinical/borderline hypothyroidism
- They have congenital hypothyroidism
- Any other disease or disorder involving the thyroid gland

Hashimoto's or Autoimmune Hypothyroidism

Around 90% of those with hypothyroidism have Hashimoto's Thyroiditis as the cause for it. Hashimoto's is an autoimmune disease which manifests as the body attacking and destroying its own thyroid gland, causing hypothyroidism as the thyroid loses function and the ability to produce adequate thyroid hormone.

If they do have Hashimoto's, the patient is known to have autoimmune hypothyroidism, meaning they actually have two forms of thyroid disease.

However, there are some people who can have Hashimoto's without losing much thyroid function, for example, if they catch the autoimmune disease early enough that it hasn't caused much damage to their thyroid gland yet, and so do not have hypothyroidism or an underactive thyroid. This is somewhat rare as most people only start to have symptoms of Hashimoto's and hypothyroidism once a lot of damage to the thyroid has already been done and thyroid hormone replacement medication tends to be needed for life by this point. Hashimoto's isn't curable but is manageable.

So, the term 'Hashimoto's' or 'Autoimmune Hypothyroidism' is suitable for:

- Those with Hashimoto's Thyroiditis, as shown by positive thyroid antibodies (TpoAB and TgAB) whether they also have hypothyroidism as a result of it or not

What is Hypothyroidism?

Hypothyroidism is a condition resulting from low thyroid hormone levels, due to the thyroid gland, located at the front of your neck, not creating enough. The five thyroid hormones are: T1, T2, T3, T4 and Calcitonin. The most important being T3 and T4, with T3 being the active thyroid hormone (what is used by cells for immediate energy and bodily functions) and T4 the stored hormone (which is often converted into T3 later on, when needed).

These hormones are needed for every process, every cell and every function in the body, so when they go wrong i.e. are too low, a lot of other stuff can go wrong too.

This can include:

- Metabolic function
- Sensitivity to heat and cold
- Muscle/joint aches and pains, cramps and weakness
- Fatigue
- Adrenal problems
- Vitamin deficiencies
- Weight gain and inability to lose weight
- Constipation and/or wind often
- Depression, anxiety and other mental health difficulties
- Slow movements, speech and thoughts
- Itchy and sore scalp
- Poor appetite
- Dry and tight feeling skin
- Brittle hair and nails
- Loss of libido (sex drive)
- Pain, numbness and a tingling sensation in the hand and fingers
- Numbness in limbs
- Period problems
- Brain fog/confusion/memory problems
- Migraines
- Hoarse voice
- A puffy-looking face
- Thinned or partly missing eyebrows

- A slow heart rate or one that increases more so than a healthy person's, after physical activity (e.g. after walking up the stairs or emptying the washing machine)
- Hearing loss
- Anaemia
- Poor stamina
- Feeling weak
- The need to nap more than others
- Long recovery period after any activity
- Inability to exercise, or withstand certain exercises
- Diagnosis of Chronic Fatigue Syndrome
- Being overly emotional
- Poor circulation
- High or rising cholesterol
- Acid reflux
- IBS
- Hair loss
- Easy bruising
- Swollen legs that impede walking
- Shin splints
- Difficulty standing on feet
- Fertility issues

Do any of these sound like the person you know with hypothyroidism? Perhaps a lightbulb has just switched on and connections between the person you see and know and their thyroid condition have wired up.

Does your friend, family member or spouse with hypothyroidism feel very tired a lot of the time? Do they need to rest or nap often?

Are they often cold and need a blanket in the evenings or a hot water bottle at night?

Did they start to feel unwell a while ago and have never quite been the same since?

Many thyroid patients find that they have their own combination of this long list of symptoms or even experience something not shown here. In fact, this list is by no means exhaustive; as part of my advocacy, I'm always hearing about new symptoms of hypothyroidism. As thyroid hormone is required for every cell and every function in the body, when we don't have enough of them, the effects can be far-reaching.

Adam's Insights

As I found with Rachel, it can really be any combination of these symptoms and what I want to stress is that the number of symptoms the thyroid patient in your life may have doesn't necessarily equate to how bad they feel. For example, one symptom doesn't mean that they only feel mildly unwell, or that a hundred of them means they're very ill. They can also be affected by different symptoms on different days.

I saw Rachel be told by doctors that her hypothyroidism was 'only mild' (borderline) yet she had twenty plus symptoms and it was incredibly hard to see someone I love being told that they are 'only mildly' hypothyroid, despite the devastating issues she was going through.

I've also witnessed Rachel talk to thyroid patients who only present a few symptoms, yet they're struggling to hold down their job and do the 'normal' things required from them. We have seen just how upsetting this can be for them, and the ones around them. An important thing I've learnt over the last few years is just how unique each person's experience with hypothyroidism can be and how they must be treated as the individual they are too.

Sit down with the thyroid patient in your life and have an honest conversation about how they're doing. Have them list all the symptoms they're currently experiencing and discuss how this is making them feel and how it is impacting their day to day life. Understanding the symptoms that they're showing today or have had in the past will help you both understand this condition.

The main purpose of thyroid hormone is to ensure that the metabolism is running properly, with the metabolism's job being to produce heat and fuel. Heat to keep us warm and fuel to give us energy. If we don't have enough of these thyroid hormones, our metabolism won't work properly and so can't provide us with adequate heat and fuel. Therefore, people with hypothyroidism can have a slow metabolism, so may also have symptoms associated with this, such as cold intolerance (from the lack of heat made) and extreme tiredness and weight gain (from the lack of calories burned to make energy).

Hypothyroidism affects its host differently, with some people reporting taking their medication each day and feeling fine, whereas other patients reporting that their medication does not help them, or that it did at one time, but not anymore.

Ultimately, once thyroid levels are optimal and the thyroid condition is being optimally treated, most symptoms should start to disappear, but support for other possible problems like vitamin deficiencies, other health conditions and adrenal dysfunction for example, will need to be in place until they recover, too. It is a multifaceted disease and many people with hypothyroidism and on medication still feel unwell. Despite their doctor telling them they just need to take one pill a day and they'll be fine.

Adam's Insights

Do not be surprised to find that your loved one may develop other conditions after/during their time being hypothyroid. This can be daunting and frustrating for everyone, but knowing that it could be a possibility helps.

What Are Optimal Thyroid Levels?

I always encourage thyroid patients to get thyroid test results printed off, for ease of reference and comparison as they move forward in their health.

Optimal thyroid levels refer to test results that align with the thyroid patient feeling optimally well. Therefore, it is not just about falling within a medical range (the numbers shown in brackets besides a test result), but aiming for optimal places within said range.

Many thyroid advocacies, progressive and functional medicine practitioners agree that a TSH less than 2 or 2.5, a Free T3 in the top quarter of the range, with a Free T4 mid-range or a little higher is considered optimal. There are also studies demonstrating that these levels may be preferable, too. [2][3][4][5]

Since most people with thyroid conditions didn't have their thyroid levels tested before developing it, we often do not know what their levels were when they felt well. So, it is crucial that they work with a doctor to find where their own individual optimal levels are.

Different Medication Options

Something else we should be aware of is that various thyroid medication options exist. Standard medication prescribed for hypothyroidism is usually synthetic T4-only medication such as Levothyroxine or Synthroid, but this doesn't eliminate symptoms and raise all levels to 'optimal' in every thyroid patient.

As we discussed previously, the thyroid gland produces five hormones, T1, T2, T3, T4 and Calcitonin, with T3 and T4 being the most important and produced in the highest quantities. With T4 being the stored hormone and T3 being the active hormone, the one that is used in our bodily functions and the one which we rely on to feel and function well. A fully functioning thyroid gland is designed to convert the stored hormone (T4) into the active hormone (T3). It is understandable that we require adequate levels of both, though perhaps most importantly T3, to feel healthy.

T4-only medications are just that. They only contain T4 and rely on the body to convert enough of this to T3. Some people do not convert adequately and so this is where taking a T3 containing medication may improve their health drastically.

Adam's Insights

Something I didn't realise until we were well into Rachel's thyroid journey is how thyroid medication can change over time. I soon adapted to not expect the type of medication or even the dosage, to stay the same forever. Being fixed on the same dose of thyroid medication for life is unusual. As a result, hypothyroidism needs to be monitored and kept on top of and with this can come changes in dosage, but also type of medication, if the one they're on just doesn't seem to be helping anymore.

The type of medication and dosage your loved one is put on initially probably won't be the same ten years down the line, after a big flare up in their health or even during or after a pregnancy.

As a spouse of a thyroid patient, I always say that I feel I'm in quite a unique position to provide an outside perspective and notice when Rachel is slowing down or struggling more so than usual. I often know when she needs a dosage adjustment before she does.

As is human nature, a lot of people will try to battle through a rough patch in their health, but ultimately I've known when Rachel's thyroid levels are off because it changes her personality, her moods, what she is able to do and even how happy we are as a couple. I can see when she's pushing herself too far, as well.

The loved ones of thyroid patients are in a really strong position to help them keep on top of this and doing so will reinforce you working together as a team in their health management, reinforcing understanding in your relationship too.

Has your loved one been particularly tired recently? Without changing their routine or what is 'normal'? This can be a sign that their thyroid levels and medication may need a review.

As a thyroid advocate, I often describe having hypothyroidism and getting better as like piecing together a big jigsaw puzzle. The experience of recovering your health can differ from person to person, with the jigsaw pieces each person needs to slot back in to place being individual to them. These can include a change in type of thyroid medication, dietary adjustments, sex hormone imbalances, gut health, supplements and so much more. Often, thyroid medication is just one piece of the puzzle. It may not solve all symptoms.

Adam's Insights

A lot of this can seem quite scary and overwhelming, for both you and your loved one. However, the amount of online information and resources about hypothyroidism is vast and thyroid conditions are a lot more common than you probably realise. One of the most impactful symptoms Rachel had was 'brain fog'. This fogginess of thought meant that holding simple conversations, Rachel learning new things and remembering what to pick up for the weekly shopping became hard. Learning even *some* information on hypothyroidism will take some of the burden of getting diagnosed off your loved one. Learning what this condition means to both of you will make things easier.

When Rachel first came home and told me she had just been diagnosed with a condition for which she would be on medication for life, I panicked. I thought *"if she's going to be on lifelong medication, does that mean it's a terminal illness? What does this mean for us?"*

When she explained that it was a chronic health condition, I was still none the wiser. Understanding that a chronic illness typically means a lifelong health condition and one that is truly individual, helped.

What Causes Hypothyroidism?

Hashimoto's Thyroiditis: The Most Common Cause for Hypothyroidism

Hashimoto's Disease is responsible for around 90% of Hypothyroidism cases. As touched on previously, it is an autoimmune disease that causes the body to attack and destroy its own thyroid gland, leading to hypothyroidism as the thyroid begins to dysfunction (lose ability to produce as much thyroid hormone as it should) from the damage caused.

As time goes by, if this autoimmune disease is not well controlled, the body continues to destroy the thyroid, causing a loss of function, which can lead to test results getting gradually worse, meaning further increases in thyroid medication dosage or the initial diagnosis of hypothyroidism.

Triggers for Hashimoto's are widely said to include adrenal dysfunction, chronic stress, toxins, poor diet, food sensitivities, viral infections, vitamin deficiencies, leaky gut, iodine deficiency, use of contraceptive pills, a blow to the immune system such as severe illness or pregnancy, and more.

There is no cure for Hashimoto's but it can be controlled and managed to limit further destruction of thyroid function and worsening thyroid hormone levels. I discuss how it can be controlled in my first book, *Be Your Own Thyroid Advocate*, however, as a book speaking to the friends and family of a thyroid patient this time around, focusing on supporting relationships rather than implementing health interventions, I feel that in-depth information on thyroid patient health interventions does not fit in naturally here. You can find more in-depth information on interventions for getting thyroid health back on track on my website or in my first book, but we will of course touch on it lightly throughout *You, Me and Hypothyroidism*.

Genetics

The thyroid gland may not develop properly at birth, known as congenital hypothyroidism. This is a condition resulting from an absent or underdeveloped thyroid gland, or one that has developed but cannot make enough thyroid hormone. For some babies, their thyroid gland does not form in its normal position in the neck. In others, the gland does not develop at all. And for others, it is simply just underdeveloped. About 3,000 children a year are born with congenital hypothyroidism in the UK.[6]

The thyroid gland may also fail later on in life, which is more common and it appears that having Down Syndrome also increases the risk of having accompanying hypothyroidism.

Radioactive Iodine Therapy and Radiation

A treatment often used for hyperthyroidism (an overactive thyroid) or certain cancers, Radioactive Iodine Therapy, often results in hypothyroidism, where the thyroid is permanently disabled from working at all or working less than it used to.

Surgery

Surgery to remove the thyroid gland often leads to hypothyroidism. If only part of the thyroid is removed, the remaining may still be able to produce enough thyroid hormone alone, but often doesn't, so medication for life can be needed to replace the hormones that are missing.

The Environment

Toxins are all around us. Chlorine and Fluoride are big ones for thyroid disease, as well as Mercury. Many people have mercury in their dental fillings, which have been said to contribute to hypothyroidism, due to the way it can affect selenium levels, with selenium being vital to thyroid function.

Dr Barry Durrant-Peatfield also explains in his book *Your Thyroid and how to keep it healthy.. The Great Thyroid Scandal and How to Survive it*, how high dosage cortisones, given for asthma and rheumatoid arthritis for example, such as dioxins and PCBs, can remain in the body for a long time affect the liver, reproductive processes, immune system, adrenals and thyroid function.

Other medications such as those for heart conditions, cancer, psychiatric conditions, lithium etc. can also affect thyroid function. Many functional medicine practitioners and doctors such as Dr Datis Kharrazian and Dr Jolene Brighten, state that too much oestrogen, often caused by taking the contraceptive pill, can lead to hypothyroidism. Contraceptive pills can also deplete vitamins and nutrients, leading to deficiencies that increase thyroid hormones binding meaning that less is available for use by cells.

Excess oestrogen can also affect how much thyroid hormone is used by the body.

Deficiencies

Deficiencies in certain vitamins, minerals and nutrients can also lead to hypothyroidism. Iodine is a well-recognised one, as adequate iodine is needed for proper thyroid function. It promotes energy and the conversion of T4 to T3, so low levels of it can cause low levels of thyroid hormone.

Adrenal Dysfunction

A failing thyroid gland can cause the adrenal glands to become stressed and fatigued. But it is also speculated to work the other way around, too.

'Adrenal Fatigue' (though it is more accurately referred to as hypothalamic-pituitary axis dysfunction) is, in Thyroid Pharmacist Izabella Wentz's experience, present in 90% of those with autoimmune hypothyroidism. [7]

The adrenal glands, which sit atop the kidneys, are responsible for producing hormones in relation to stress, such as the hormone cortisol. There are two well-recognised conditions in medicine, in association with extreme dysfunctioning of the adrenal glands: Addison's, which is a long-term condition whereby the adrenal glands do not produce enough cortisol and Cushing's, which is the opposite; where the adrenals produce often dangerously high levels of the hormone.

Adrenal fatigue is a condition where the adrenal glands produce too much or too little cortisol, though not to the extent of Cushing's or Addison's Disease, but abnormal enough that it can cause symptoms and issues. It works on the idea that there is a scale rather than just extremes.

Adrenal fatigue can include elevated, lowered or mixed levels of cortisol. Thousands of people report symptoms and problems, especially thyroid related, with adrenal fatigue, which resolve once cortisol levels are back within 'normal ranges'. Symptoms of adrenal fatigue are similar to thyroid symptoms.

I have included a book by Dr. Wilson, concerning adrenal fatigue, in the list at the back of this book.

Treating underlying causes for adrenal fatigue, e.g. dietary issues/sensitivities, sex hormone imbalances low thyroid hormone levels, exercise and stress, are all involved in fixing the adrenal dysfunction that exists. Dysfunctional adrenal glands can result in thyroid hormone levels looking 'normal' but with ongoing symptoms and issues. Testing is usually via a 24 hour, four-point saliva test.

Adam's Insights

Once Rachel had worked on getting her thyroid levels in check, the next thing we focused on was the Adrenal Dysfunction. It's often hard to distinguish between which are hypothyroid symptoms and which are adrenal symptoms. Understanding the differences and that Adrenal Fatigue or other factors could be the thing holding back your loved one's recovery can help unlock the path to getting back to 'normal'.

Trauma

Direct damage such as whiplash, being roughly handled around the throat, hitting your chin on the dashboard in a car accident etc. can understandably lead to a damaged thyroid gland and thus, affect its output of hormones.

Pregnancy

As pregnancy is stressful on the body, it can induce hypothyroidism. For some women, it comes to surface during pregnancy, but it is after pregnancy that a lot are diagnosed. Some recover after a month or two, but many are left with hypothyroidism for the rest of their lives.

During pregnancy, the body goes through many hormonal changes and the immune system makes adjustments in order to preserve the foetus and not reject it as a foreign invader. The Th-1 suppression ends after birth and this causes the immune system to surge. If it is already unstable, then this can trigger the start of Hashimoto's Thyroiditis.

Central Hypothyroidism

Although rare, if something is wrong with the pituitary gland, this can interfere with the production of thyroid hormones. The pituitary gland produces TSH, which tells the thyroid how much hormones it should make and release. If something is wrong with the pituitary gland, then thyroid hormone production and release will be affected, causing hypothyroidism.

A similar problem can be of the hypothalamus too. Although rare, hypothyroidism can occur if the hypothalamus, situated in the brain, does not produce enough TRH, which tells the pituitary to release TSH.

Adam's Insights

As a loved one, try not to get too hung up on the why's or what's in terms of what lead them to develop hypothyroidism. I worry that a feeling of blame may be placed on the thyroid patient, when in reality, they are of course not at fault for having a thyroid condition.

Searching for answers when the true cause of hypothyroidism and Hashimoto's can often not be found isn't productive. As her partner, I was often quick to 'solutionize' when Rachel was first diagnosed. I wanted to find a 'fix' or something that could make things better faster, but I assure you that this way of thinking, whilst well-meant, will often lead to conflict and your loved one feeling misunderstood. Listening to them is often all your loved one needs right now and spending too much time in the past instead of focusing on what you can do now, in the present, can be more unproductive than productive.

Chapter 3: Getting the Most Out of Medical Appointments

"Support each other, as together you are the best team." - Adam Gask

There are several occasions when your presence at appointments concerning your loved one's thyroid condition will be much appreciated. And perhaps even necessary for being listened to and moving forward in getting their health back on track.

Many people with hypothyroidism feel unheard by their doctors, put down or doubted. The words 'hypochondriac' and "It's all in your head" are unfortunately common place. It is understandable therefore that the person you know with hypothyroidism may feel anxious and worried about upcoming appointments, followed by feeling frustrated and disappointed afterwards.

To help the thyroid patient in your life get the most out of their medical appointments, you can support them in a few ways:

Go to Appointments with Them

The main thing you can do in supporting them with medical appointments is by attending them with your loved one. They'll appreciate the support and from personal experience, your presence will likely also validate what they're saying.

Appointments where Adam has attended with me always seem to go smoother and have better outcomes, as he contributes to what is said and adds another point of view to the situation. I always feel taken more seriously when I'm accompanied by someone else as it is harder for the doctor to blow off my concerns when someone else is there backing them up, too.

It doesn't have to be a romantic partner. A friend or family member can also be hugely helpful.

Adam's Insights

Being able to chime in with how I see Rachel's health affecting her quality of life is always very valuable to a medical appointment. I can provide a different perspective and, when delivered in a matter of fact way, can help medical professionals feel like the impact that hypothyroidism is having on Rachel's health is more than an inconvenience. It can feel as if reiterating the struggles Rachel has, has a greater influence on the conversation than her personal experiences and frustrations. I have experienced appointments where Rachel has often forgotten key things she has been planning to say for weeks prior during the short time she gets to speak to a medical professional, but by being in the room I was able to help prompt her with things she wanted to say, rather than her regretting not saying anything later on.

The next time you accompany an appointment with the thyroid patient in your life, consider jotting down a few examples of how you see them struggling and mention them to the doctor. Be prepared to be quizzed yourself too; in some bizarre appointments I have had medical professionals totally ignore my input and get agitated with my comments, until they ask how long we have been together. Once confirming I am a long-term partner (one that has seen Rachel before and after being diagnosed with hypothyroidism), they seem to value my comments more than hers! Do not underestimate the influence your thoughts can have; they can be the deciding factor in a successful vs unsuccessful appointment for you both.

Help Them Plan

If your loved one has also been reading, doing research and collecting information regarding thyroid treatment and management - for example regarding other thyroid medication options, further testing they may benefit from or suspected vitamin deficiencies, help them prepare any supporting materials by printing out information on studies and research, making notes and highlighting important parts and take it along.

It may also be helpful for you to take an active part in researching and compiling information too. Thyroid fatigue and brain fog can make it difficult to concentrate, retain and process information. Please see a list of websites and literature for recommended reading at the back of this book.

Adam's Insights

As loved ones, we must try to understand how scary it can be for the thyroid patients in our lives to go in to a doctor and open up about their problems, all the while knowing that you may not even be believed. I've seen just how tiring it has been on Rachel, both before, during and after appointments. As someone who has only ever visited the doctor for more 'routine' appointments I never had an instance where I felt like a doctor might not believe me. In fact, I found it hard to believe this to ever be the case. When Rachel mentioned after an appointment I didn't attend with her that she felt ignored, my initial reaction was one to defend the medical professional. But having been through that process with her, it can be a common occurrence, one that as loved ones we must accept and support.

If they are anxious before going to an appointment, the best thing you can do is try to be as understanding as possible. Can you help to prepare them? Or plan for what you might do afterwards? Could you plan to spend some time after an appointment on something that is totally different and unrelated to their health?

Can you help them to practise what they want to say to the doctor beforehand, in order to help them feel more confident? Whilst in the doctor's office, would it help if you prompted them so they don't forget to mention all points? This can help to ensure these opportunities aren't lost.

Presentation and Body Language

Ensure your loved one leads the appointment and wait for natural breaks in conversation or for prompts from them or the doctor, before speaking.

Adam's Insights

In the rush of emotions at a medical appointment, your loved one may feel brain fogged, confused and overwhelmed. So, ensure you listen to everything discussed too. Be their champion. You might be the one who retains the important information said and will need to relay this back to your loved one at a later date.

You also want to support what they're saying, so make sure to wait for natural breaks before speaking so as not to speak over them or appear to be patronising. Continue to support them by helping them be independent and assertive. Remain matter of fact, especially if your loved one is emotional, as it will help the medical professional see that what is being discussed isn't being blown out of proportion.

Prepare Them for Undesirable Outcomes

It's always possible that despite preparing for a medical appointment very thoroughly, the outcome may not be as expected or as hoped. Discuss the outcome they're hoping for ahead of time, but also speak about the less desirable ones and be prepared to hear them, too. Consider reactions to these and if possible, come up with an action plan for them too.

For example, if the aim of the appointment is to ask for more comprehensive thyroid testing because they've only ever had TSH tested before, and the doctor refuses, your plan B could be to order the tests yourself by using an online laboratory service.

If your loved one is asking their doctor to test them for Coeliac Disease or gluten sensitivity as they believe gluten is making their symptoms worse, but the doctor says "No", they could instead plan to determine if they have an adverse effect to gluten by simply removing it from their diet for a month or two instead.

Adam's Insights

Planning for the best and worst outcomes from medical appointments will protect you from being blindsided about what to do next. The hypothyroid patient might be particularly emotional and by being the calming influence, you can help them take their next step.

Consider Time Before and After the Appointment

Adam's Insights

There have been times in the past where I've known Rachel has an important medical appointment coming up and over time, I've learnt to keep our schedule around it empty. I make sure to limit our social commitments and focus on us having the breathing space to either spend some time together or for Rachel to take some time to reflect and chill out.

It helps to know that you're not rushing, following these appointments and that you can sit and talk about how you each felt it went and what actions you will be taking forward. Allow for this to take some time, not everyone will want to make big decisions or talk in detail about the future, it can be scary for everyone. They might have had this appointment on their mind for a long time and will want a mental break before carrying on.

If the appointment goes badly, it may not be a good idea to have commitments they then have to go on to do. Time to process for everyone is important.

I have also learnt over the years which tips and tricks help cheer Rachel up after a bad medical appointment. Whether I keep a hidden bar of chocolate, offer her a foot massage, encourage her to get lost in a novel or stick our favourite TV boxset on, it can make such a difference in keeping those lines of communication between us both open. The last thing you want is for them to start closing you off. Let them know you support them.

Closing Thoughts

Adam's Insights

As a loved one of someone with hypothyroidism, and from personal experience, I know how big a role you can play at medical appointments. As Rachel has mentioned, the phrases 'you're just a hypochondriac' and 'It's all in your head' can really come to the fore. But accompanying Rachel to her medical appointments has meant she's been taken more seriously and I can't say a doctor has ever uttered those words when I am in the room.

By me simply being there, it adds so much credibility and unfortunately, I've experienced the fact that as a man accompanying a woman to (most often) a male doctor's office, I am often seen as someone who adds more credibility to what she's already telling them. And that doesn't feel right at all. Why should I have more validity on how her health is? Not the patient?

In fact, research has indicated that medical professionals are more likely to interpret men's symptoms as biological and women's symptoms as psychosocial. Implying that a lot of women's symptoms are a result of a mental, rather than physical, illness. Or simply all in their head. This isn't acceptable, but something that does happen. Preparing for this and knowing that if you're lucky to have this 'superpower' (the mystical 'Y' chromosome) you can leverage this to have added effect so that your loved one is listened to properly.

The amount of times where Rachel has seen a doctor once and not had a productive conversation with them, so we go in together the next day and have a completely different outcome, despite saying the same things, is astounding.

Chapter 4: Understanding How Your Loved One's Energy Levels Work

"If you love someone, let them nap." - Rachel Hill, The Invisible Hypothyroidism

The Spoon Theory

Adam describes the moment that I shared the simple analogy of The Spoon Theory with him, as a light bulb being switched on. It made it easier for him to understand how my energy levels and depletions worked.

The spoon theory is a metaphor that those with a disability, chronic illness or disease, often use to explain the reduced amount of energy available for activities of daily living and tasks. A Spoonie is someone with a health condition that needs to watch their 'spoons'. Spoons are their unit of energy.

The spoon theory, created by Christine Miserandino, explains how those living with disability or chronic illness can have a limited amount of energy.[8] This can be in day to day living or just during thyroid flare ups. The idea is that many people with a disability or chronic illness must carefully plan their daily activities in order to use their energy wisely, whilst most people with better health or who do not have a disability, do not need to worry about running out of energy.

'Spoons' are a unit of measurement used to track how much energy a person has throughout the day. Imagine that you start the day with a certain number of 'spoons'. You need to get through the day without using them all too early on. Yet each activity requires a certain number of spoons, such as having a shower, walking to work, making dinner etc. and

39

spoons will only be replaced when you rest. If you run out of spoons, you have no choice but to rest until they are replenished.

For example, you could start each day with ten spoons and tasks such as showering or bathing require two spoons, and walking for half an hour requires six. Or four. Or even one. Different tasks can use different amounts of energy for different people.

Those of us with limited energy reserves have to work out which activities we can afford to do each day, so as not to run out of spoons (energy) and be left exhausted.

You can also end up going in to the next day's allocation of spoons by overexerting yourself and then take longer to replenish them. You can build up a spoon debt which must be repaid at some point.

As other people without a disability or chronic illness often do not feel the impact of spending spoons for mundane tasks such as bathing and getting dressed, they may not realise the amount of energy used by those who *do* need to plan their energy usage just to get through the day. They do not tend to have a limited amount of energy, as most daily tasks could never get close to exhausting them, unlike those with hypothyroidism for example.

However, even those who have their hypothyroidism well-managed can be more at risk of over exhausting and expecting too much of themselves, compared to others. We can also go through periods of flare ups in thyroid symptoms.

As someone who knows a Spoonie, you should be aware of how they manage their energy levels and look for signs that they may be doing *too much*. Offering to help with certain tasks and saving them some spoons can mean they are actually able to do more with you.

Adam taking on more of the housework for example has meant that I don't run out of energy as quickly as I used to, which meant I would nap a lot. Instead, now I have more energy or 'spoons', thanks to him helping me protect them and use them more wisely. I can now spend more time with him doing the things we love instead of recuperating constantly.

Adam's Insights

As someone who has never experienced the feeling of completely running out of energy, I can only confirm what it is not like. The concept of tasks taking up a chunk of someone's total daily energy was a profound moment. When I have lots to do, I of course get tired, but I might take a break, do something else and then power through. This simply isn't possible for a lot of people with a chronic illness; there really is an upper limit to what they can do.

Yes, I've experienced perhaps drinking a tad too much the night before and feeling worn out the following day. I've experienced colds and a bad night's sleep. I completed a marathon a few years ago. But none of these have been comparable to how Rachel is on a 'low spoon day'. Understanding The Spoon Theory and essentially how her energy levels work as a thyroid patient, has been a key part of strengthening our relationship. I now know and understand that she does sometimes have a limited amount of energy from day to day, and not limitless, like myself.

On her worst days with hypothyroidism, she could run out of energy by the afternoon on a Saturday and at first I just didn't understand why. After all, we hadn't done much.

I'd get in from work and find her asleep on the sofa, in her coat as she didn't even have the energy to remove it before lying down. But we had both been at work all day and I felt fine. So why didn't she? This can easily cause a strain between you, as what is a real lack of available energy can be misinterpreted as laziness.

Those mundane, everyday tasks we non-spoonies don't think about such as showering, walking ten minutes to the shops or cooking dinner, are often traded for 'spoons' in their situation. It's not laziness, trust me. I'm married to a very motivated, determined woman that used to be a morning person and always on the go, before her hypothyroidism diagnosis.

Over time, I have taken on more in the way I help out around the house and taken more of the initiative, due to this helpful 'spoon' analogy. You learn to read how many 'spoons' your loved one has left and once you understand that concept, your relationship with them starts to feel like it is back in your control again. If we have a restful morning, then I know Rachel will likely have enough energy to go out in the evening. If I can see she's doing well on energy at lunchtime then we can go out for a long walk without depleting her spoons. This balance and understanding is key.

We like to go out for walks every day, whether it's at lunchtime on the weekends or in the evenings on work days. I can often gauge how long a walk we should be taking by reading Rachel's energy levels. We generally aim for an average of 45-minutes, but alter this depending on her spoon reserves. The last thing I want is for her to overdo it, but by being aware of this, we have a more fulfilling time together.

The way I see hypothyroidism on low energy days is like this: it is like a car running out of fuel. You can't 'will it' to move if there's no fuel in it. It took me a while to understand that you can apply this analogy to a health condition like hypothyroidism. On days where your loved one has literally crashed and run out of energy, be careful not to imply that they could still do things 'if only they tried hard enough'. You wouldn't expect a car that has no fuel in it to keep going. No amount of 'willing' will get it down the street.

It also takes time for someone with a chronic illness to set their scale, to understand themselves just how many spoons they have on a 'good' day, how many are used in day to day tasks and how different things can increase or decrease their daily total. Things like a bad night's sleep or having a bubble bath after work can make a huge impact, both negatively and positively on this figure.

By understanding capabilities, we can manage expectations and feel more satisfied.

Thyroid Flare Ups

A flare up is defined by an increase in symptoms of hypothyroidism. A flare up can last anywhere from a few days to a few weeks. Symptoms can differ from person to person, though the most commonly reported in a flare up are:

- Increased fatigue
- Heaviness (as if your body is being weighed down)
- Worsened mental health
- Brain fog
- Migraines
- Flu-like symptoms (aches and pains)
- Switching between feeling really cold and really hot

What Causes a Flare Up?

What causes a flare up is very much individual to each thyroid patient, but these are the most commonly reported:

- Drinking alcohol
- Eating poorly (such as a lot of sugary or processed food, not giving the body good nutrition)
- Consuming a known food allergen or sensitivity (such as gluten, dairy, soy etc.)
- Overexertion (mentally and/or physically) - ignoring 'spoon usage'
- Stress
- Not sticking to a good sleep routine

- Viral, bacterial, fungal etc. infections
- Being on your period or due to start on your period (hormonal fluctuations)
- Pregnancy

How Can I Help in a Flare Up?

First and foremost, it is important to say that if anyone is feeling incredibly unwell, then they should always see their doctor in case something more serious is going on.

However, the best thing you can do when supporting someone going through a thyroid flare up, is by encouraging them to rest and recuperate. This may include them needing to take time off work, or if this isn't viable, limiting how much their work impedes their recovery from a flare up. For example, this could include them seeking permission to work from home, working altered hours until the flare up has passed, replacing walking to and from work with transport, or otherwise speaking to the line manager about suitable adjustments.

If making changes surrounding their work isn't an option, you can still support them in recuperating outside of work as much as possible. Help them to limit how much unnecessary activity they do and maximise resting and recuperation time.

Looking at the list of triggers above, you can use these to also guide you, such as encouraging them to think about nutrition, avoiding stress, keeping warm, drinking plenty of water and getting plenty of sleep/rest.

It is perfectly normal to expect flare ups in symptoms from time to time and as you experience them more often, you will become more accustomed to how you can help them through it.

A Note from Rachel's Friend Liz

"Seeing a friend (now family since she married Adam, my cousin) go through a flare up day without knowing what to do was a hard sight to see. Rachel woke up feeling stiff and tired and I witnessed her having a panic attack as she felt so unwell. Luckily, Adam was there too and I was able to watch how he handled it and take his guidance on what I could do to help. Following this, I managed to help calm Rachel down and talk her through it. After doing that, I ran her a bath and as she soaked in it, we spoke about everyday things. It seemed to help and I was glad.

Since Rachel has gone gluten-free for her thyroid health, I have also taken it upon myself to learn what ingredients I am looking for so I can accommodate her needs and help her stay on top of feeling good and limiting flare up days."

Adam's Insights

In a flare up, if you can try different things to figure out what works for your loved one as well as openly asking them how you can help, it can build a mutual understanding. If Rachel is particularly cold, despite already placing her under a duvet and hugging a hot water bottle, I'll put the heating on or make her another hot water bottle. Asking her at the time hasn't always been easy, so we regularly check in on her non-flare days to understand what helps her best.

In terms of trying to keep her stress levels low, I also tend to take stock of any tasks that need doing.

If we were planning to do a grocery shop, I'll likely go on my own while she rests at home, or if there are a few jobs around the house, I'll crack on with these so they're one less thing she has to worry about.

However, she may prefer that I sit and spend time with her instead, so I often gauge what is best on that day. This can be a hard balance to find, and sometimes one that I don't get right, but learning what works and doesn't work means I get better at handling her flare ups each and every time.

What is it that you can implement to help? Is it a foot soak? A leg massage? Their favourite dinner? A film that always makes them laugh? Would it help if you helped them get ready? Or do they prefer to simply have time on their own?

You as the loved one may well be the person in their circle who understands how they're affected by a flare up best. Could you speak to those around you and help to make them more aware of how your loved one is affected? If it also affects social plans, you may need to explain to people why you're having to pull out of attending. This can be hard or awkward at times, but often a lot less awkward than for your loved one. Remember, they often feel incredibly guilty at missing out on events due to their illness, so try not to add to this when it happens.

Chapter 5: Words of Support

"Never judge people. You never know what it took for them to face the day today." - Rachel Hill, The Invisible Hypothyroidism

What Not to Say to Someone with Hypothyroidism

The below comments can cause people living with hypothyroidism to feel very alone, misunderstood, misjudged and avoid turning to people for help and support in the future, so they can be very detrimental.

This list hasn't been created to moan at you, the loved one, but to educate you so that you're able to help the thyroid patient in your life, as the support you can provide will aid their recovery a lot.

You may even be as shocked to hear these as we often are!

1. "You just need a good night's sleep."

Unfortunately, this just isn't how it works. Believe us, we've tried sleeping lots and we're not cured yet! And if you live with someone with hypothyroidism, you've probably noticed how much they sleep and how little difference it seems to make. In fact, we're so fatigued that we often sleep more than anyone else we know. It's frustrating!

Thyroid hormone directly controls and affects energy levels, which means that fatigue is one of the most commonly complained of symptoms with the condition. We are easily tired and often feel tired all the time, scarcely waking up feeling refreshed. The best way I can describe it is *every-second-*

I'm-consciously-having-to-keep-each-eyelid-open tired. It's *I'm-scared-to-blink-or-I'll-fall-asleep* tired. It's exhaustion past the point of exhaustion.

2. "You've got medicine now, so you must be fine."

Not necessarily and this is a very big misconception. Unfortunately, it can take months or even years for people to get their thyroid medication right.

Since a lot of doctors aren't usually very helpful when it comes to trying different medication options to see what works for each patient, it can be a real upwards battle at times. Most tend to have a 'one medication works for all' approach which is very unhelpful. And even when we do get our thyroid medication right, we can also have other conditions that have developed because of the thyroid not being adequately treated for quite some time.

This includes vitamin deficiencies, adrenal problems, mental health conditions and digestive issues to name just a few. So, don't just assume we're OK once we're put on thyroid medication, as it's usually just the beginning! We're happy to talk to you about how we're doing and how our current medication is working.

Adam's Insights

If you've never had a chronic illness, it can be easy to think "The doctor has said that you just need to take this medication each day and you'll be fine, so you should be fine." But everyone is different, so we cannot apply this across the board. Medication can also take time to get fully integrated into the body, so give any new medication and change the time it needs to work.

3. "Be patient."

Being told to give the thyroid medication time to work can be frustrating. If we become a little impatient, frustrated or fed up, please bear with us. We've probably had a long battle with getting this diagnosis in the first place, so allow us to feel a little impatient. Don't you feel impatient waiting for the *us* you remember before hypothyroidism, to fully return?

Adam's Insights

I know I felt impatient waiting for the Rachel I fell in love with and had been with for so long, to finally return. However, you being impatient doesn't get them back to good health any sooner. It may just make things more strained.

In those early days, I learnt to take each day as it came instead of focusing on 'the goal' of resuming our lives before the diagnosis.

4. "Just eat less and exercise more!"

As the metabolism is often slowed in hypothyroidism, we can have symptoms associated with a slow metabolism, such as cold intolerance, extreme tiredness and weight gain.

We may gain weight and cannot control it. We also struggle to then lose it. Some even diet and force unhealthy exercise regimens and end up gaining more weight.

Only when our thyroid hormone levels are corrected, thus correcting our metabolic function, do we have a chance of losing excess weight and stop gaining it at all. Not to mention that most of us don't have the energy to move any more than we already do, due to the slow metabolism. Over exercising can also make you *more* hypothyroid.

Adam's Insights

Thyroid conditions are often the butt of weight jokes in society. It's easy for casual throw away comments by people around your loved one to hurt. Championing thyroid patients, when you are both with them and without them, will normalise how much of an impact thyroid disease can have on patients.

5. "It's all in your head. You just need to let it go."

My own doctor told me this when I visited him time and time again complaining of my initial thyroid medication not helping at all. Needless to say, I haven't seen that doctor since, as I was so frustrated and I found one who does now listen and has got me on the medication I need to feel well.

Adam's Insights

Unless we're in the thyroid patient's shoes, we cannot make a call on what is and isn't real. No one knows their own mind and body better than themselves.

6. "You're so hormonal!"

Please don't judge us because of our health condition. Please don't assume anything we say that you disagree with, is because our 'crazy thyroid hormones' make our moods and emotions go up and down.

We can be mad, annoyed or irritated for legitimate reasons. Maybe we're fed up with battling this health condition, but don't assume that it's just because of our thyroid hormones being off.

Adam's Insights

As a cis man, I know I should especially be careful of making such an assumption. The thyroid patient in your life is entitled to feel everything that you do too; anger, irritation or have strong opinions, without people pinning it on their health condition.

After all, we're allowed to feel those things without such comments, so why aren't they? They're still a human being under the hypothyroidism. Think carefully about such remarks. Thyroid patients also often want to feel like everyone else, and they are entitled to being human, flaws and all, too.

7. "You have this condition because of ___"

Insert 'not wearing a coat when you go out', 'your bad diet', 'not eating enough fruit and veg' etc. here. Sure, those things won't help your health, but hey, it doesn't cause thyroid problems either!

8. "The thyroid doesn't even do anything."

This not only belittles what we're going through, but it also makes you look very uninformed. Sure, I didn't even know where the thyroid gland was when I was first diagnosed! But don't assume it doesn't do anything. It actually does a lot of important stuff. The thyroid gland produces hormones needed for every process and every cell of the body, so when this goes wrong, a lot of other stuff does too!

What is Helpful to Say to Someone with Hypothyroidism

These examples are instead much more helpful and will help to strengthen your mutual understanding of the condition and experience.

1. "How are you doing?"

This simple question shows you care about us and how we're doing, and that you understand we may have a bit of a battle with getting well again. It's nice to know that someone cares and we often like to talk about it with others so we don't feel alone. Let us get things off our chest too, it's very healthy and can help us to process the change in our lives.

2. "Can I do anything to help?"

Most commonly, you won't be able to do an awful lot, but we can benefit from you helping us with errands, housework or even an ear to listen. There's not a great deal our friends, family and work colleagues can do other than to be understanding of our condition and be open minded, but we'll rarely turn down the offer of a cup of tea and a chat.

Little things mean a lot to us when we're struggling. We're really grateful for those little things.

3. "What has worked for you?"

Treating and managing hypothyroidism is often not as simple as you'd think, so we tend to have to try quite a few medications, lifestyle adjustments and more until we find what works for us. This means lots of book reading, internet searching and maybe even numerous visits to different doctors and health practitioners. It can be stressful, upsetting and really testing at times, so we'd love to share with you what we've learnt and what we're going through. It's comforting to know you understand that it isn't a simple one-cure-fits-all disease.

Adam's Insights

Taking an interest, actively listening and ensuring the thyroid patient in your life doesn't feel alone, goes a long way. But by asking this question you also build up your knowledge of the disease and what has worked in their situation. Understanding the things that do work will make your loved ones life and yours, easier.

4. "I respect your opinions/I support your choices."

Try not to dismiss us when we say that we know something isn't right, or that a particular treatment isn't working for us.

Respect us for doing our own research, and respect our opinions. Let us share our findings with you. Explore with us our ideas and acknowledge that we're entitled to our own thoughts, too. Support our choices to make changes to our health regimen if we feel it's the best thing for us. Really just try to understand and listen to us. This one is most important for partners of thyroid patients.

5. "You're looking well."

If we're looking better, brighter, happier, healthier, then let us know! It's reassuring to know that our hard work at getting ourselves better is paying off. We often lack motivation and many of us battle with mental health conditions that make it difficult to stay positive. Some praise every now and then and reminders that we're making progress can go a long way to give us the boost we need to carry on progressing in our journey to feeling better.

6. "How is the book you're reading?"

See us reading a thyroid book? A study or some research? Health magazine? A blog? Articles online maybe? Ask us what it's about, if it's any good and what we may have learnt from it. It's nice to see some interest from those around us and we'd like to share what we read with you too.

7. "You need to try another doctor."

If we're going back again and again to the same doctor and getting nowhere with feeling better, you may need to encourage us to seek out another. And another. And another.

Until we find one who will listen to us and work *with* us. We can feel intimidated or worried to make the change, but it's important for our health that we do so. Again, your support is going to be key in us making progress with our health.

Adam's Insights

It is well worth exploring different doctors as not all are the same. As well as there being different types of doctors that you can explore (conventional, naturopathic, functional etc.), doctors even differ within these types.

For example, Rachel saw a lot of different GPs on the NHS here in England and found that they differed widely in how understanding and open minded they were. We eventually found a GP that worked *with* Rachel, and that we were very thankful for, as he agreed to run comprehensive testing and support Rachel in advocating for her own health. But it took a lot of trial and error to find him. We went through most GPs at our clinic and had plans to try somewhere new.

When he unfortunately left the surgery after a few years, we made the decision to explore a private GP. Contacting local thyroid charities for lists of private practitioners, we found some and started going down this route, too. However, Rachel often became overwhelmed with taking this next step, as the whole world of private healthcare was alien to us. So, helping her to find someone and go through this new process together was crucial. After all, this change impacted the both of us.

8. "Keep on going. You will feel well again."

When this condition and all its related problems get too much for us, we need to be reminded that we must keep on going. Often, facing the idea of spending the rest of our lives feeling so unbelievably ill, is enough to make someone very depressed and/or anxious. People with hypothyroidism can get better, and although it's not always easy, it is possible. It absolutely is. They just need gentle nudges and direction on where to go, at times. Help them to help themselves.

Chapter 6: Hypothyroidism's Effects on Mental Health

"Poor mental health has the ability to completely change the person you knew."- Rachel Hill, The Invisible Hypothyroidism

Hypothyroidism often comes hand in hand with mental health conditions such as anxiety and depression. In fact, they are recognisable signs and symptoms of a thyroid condition.

In thyroid patients of all ages, many of them may be labelled with psychiatric issues such as mental health issues, when they are actually due to hormonal imbalances. For example, in one study looking at the adrenal glands it was concluded that by correcting the underlying hormonal imbalance, many patients' mental health improved, with some patients having a total reversal of psychiatric symptoms.[9]

It is therefore of paramount importance that any thyroid patient with a mental health condition be optimally treated for their hypothyroidism. Remember that 'optimal thyroid levels' are defined in Chapter 2.

Many hypothyroid patients find that their non-optimally treated hypothyroidism is brushed off as depression. Some patients do have the two separate conditions, but we also need to acknowledge that depression isn't a scapegoat for *all* symptoms left from a non-optimally treated thyroid condition.

For example, there are some symptoms of depression that can be the same as those for hypothyroidism, such as:

- Low mood
- Being slow in speech and/or movement
- Feeling more tired than normal

But equally, there are some that are not present in depression, such as:

- A puffy face
- Hair loss
- Overwhelming fatigue
- Dry skin
- Muscle weakness
- Aches and pains
- Raised blood pressure
- Raised cholesterol

These are *physical* symptoms, and not caused by something mental, but something *physically* wrong. They could well be a sign that the thyroid patient isn't adequately treated on their thyroid medication and this should be investigated.

If your loved one with hypothyroidism struggles with their mental health, you may need to advocate for them in the doctor's office to ensure they are taken seriously. Depression in particular, can devastate lives and seriously affect relationships, but if it's in fact caused by a thyroid condition, a hormonal imbalance that can be addressed rather simply, it seems silly to let it carry on wreaking its havoc.

Of course, antidepressants, anti-anxiety meds etc. can be a great help to many people and it is important not to feed the stigma that taking them is 'wrong'. I am not anti-medication, but I am pro-informed decision, which means making sure those who are thyroid patients also experiencing mental health conditions, know that addressing their endocrine health fully may well resolve their mental health complaints.

I have taken various types of antidepressants myself in the past. However, none helped me at all, which is perhaps a sign that it was due to a physical imbalance of thyroid hormone. Especially as my mental health hugely improved when optimally medicated for hypothyroidism.

The link between depression and thyroid problems is thought to involve T3, one of the hormones a healthy thyroid should be producing. Unfortunately, most of the time doctors will only prescribe T4-only medications (such as Levothyroxine/Synthroid) for hypothyroidism, so we're relying on our bodies to convert some of that into the T3 we also need, and well, that doesn't always happen so easily.

Thyroid hormone T3 has an important role in the health and optimal functioning of the brain, including: cognitive function, ability to concentrate, mood, memory, attention span, emotions and ability to cope with life's stresses. Could your loved one benefit from being on a T3-containing medication? You can tell by looking at their test results but also discussing how they're feeling on their current medication. Combining test results as well as symptoms, will create a full picture. In terms of test results, both Free T3 and T4 should be optimised, but the first step you may stumble at with this, is in confirming what has actually been tested.

If the doctor has failed to check a *full* thyroid panel, including Free T3 and Free T4, then it doesn't confirm if a conversion problem is taking place and whether someone has mental health issues caused by an inadequately treated thyroid condition. If they have all been tested, then they should be checked to see if they are optimal.

If your loved one has Hashimoto's, then it is also worth knowing that this can add additional mental health symptoms into the mix. Hashimoto's is reported to cause swings of TSH, with hyper and hypo symptoms to match. Hyperthyroid symptoms can include hyperactivity, anxiety, irritability and disturbed sleep, whilst hypothyroidism often causes fatigue and depression. Those swinging symptoms could even mimic Bipolar Disorder.

If your loved one is struggling with their mental health amidst this big thyroid puzzle, please be patient. It's difficult when your body is physically struggling, but the mental health struggles can be even more debilitating.

Breaking down at work, a reduced tolerance to stress and feeling overwhelmed over the smallest of things can take hold as we whirl around the tornado of our life being turned upside down.

Adam's Insights

Understanding when things are likely to be tough is a good way to help your hypothyroid loved one. When Rachel was having a particularly tough time with her health, I knew that the pressure of a big work meeting coming up would only make things worse. Try to help your loved one prepare for the pressures and stresses associated with work by taking an interest in their day to day work duties and what things are likely to cause them the most stress. You can then identify if things coming up, combined with a particularly tricky period of health will cause a downturn in mental health.

As well as the hormonal imbalances of physical changes happening within the body that can lead to poor mental health, the realisation that our lives will be forever different, that we may battle with our bodies on a daily basis and essentially *grieve* for our non-chronically ill lives, can be tough.

Some people grieve for months and others years. In my own experience, it has become easier with time and as I have reclaimed some of my health piece by piece. However, there is no right or wrong way to go about accepting this big change to your life that can't be undone.

Seeing Your Loved One's Mental Health Decline

Adam's Insights

It wasn't easy to see the bright, happy, busy-bee Rachel I had known for so many years, slip in to such poor mental health. I would come home from work to see her crying on the sofa, not able to smile when having an enjoyable time with friends or even be able to muster up enthusiasm for the things she used to love.

As well as depression, she also had anxiety and this showed itself mainly at work or surrounding the idea of work. Panic attacks in the morning as she got ready for work or phone calls where she could hardly breathe and needed me to help calm her down so she could return to the office - it was all a minefield to me.

When she was diagnosed with hypothyroidism, she was told to take the 'one pill a day' and she'd be fine, but I watched her only get worse as time went on, and this spread into her mental health and well-being too. Yes, the hypothyroidism affected her physical self in terms of her energy and day to day capabilities, but I was really shocked and surprised by how much it affected her mental health and just how closely tied they are. I could make an easier connection between her hypothyroidism and physical health, i.e. having less energy and sleeping more, but grasping the idea that it affected her mental health was harder.

The impact on her mental health was massive, when she wasn't optimally treated for the thyroid issue, on Levothyroxine, she was not just fighting her body but also fighting her mind, struggling with depression and anxiety on top of hypothyroidism, which seemed to amplify everything. It made things even worse.

If your loved one with hypothyroidism struggles with their mental health, you probably don't need me to say that it can really alter their personality and who they are. And that can then put a huge strain on the relationship.

When Rachel's mental health was declining, I mainly felt quite useless. With her physical health struggles, I knew I could do more around the house in order to help, but managing her mental health was daunting and something I wasn't accustomed to at all. I had to learn a lot about depression and anxiety, what made them worse for her and what made them better. For example, she has always liked being in a tidy environment, as clutter and mess makes her anxiety worse, so I became more aware of helping to maintain a tidy home. Simple but effective and it soon became second nature. Before her thyroid condition diagnosis, a messy house did frustrate her but now laying it on top of the physical health condition, it was even more of an issue. I could see that it was more frustrating to her because she had less control over doing anything about it. In my experience, lots of these little stressors can soon mount up and exacerbate each other. The small things are only the tip of the iceberg to an already rubbish week she may be having and trying to plough on through.

Over time, we have defined what we refer to as a 'wobble' in Rachel's mental health. This is when she starts to show signs of struggling to keep on top of things and mentally and emotionally wobbling. I often see a wobble coming before Rachel does and recognising this gives me the opportunity to try and diffuse it before she slips quickly into a darker place. When she 'wobbles' I tell myself to remain calm and collected as I try to steer her through it and back out to the brighter side. "It will pass", I say to us both.

What I would say to any others working their way through the mental health challenges of hypothyroidism, is to just take it step by step and day by day. Allow the person you know with this health condition to honestly explain to you, without judgement, how they feel and brainstorm some ideas on what you can both do to make some small steps back to good mental health and well-being. Be it looking in to talking therapies or counselling, focusing on eating well and getting outside more or managing expectations. Work your way through it step by step. I made the mistake of reacting at first by solutionizing, with my 'well what can I do to help?' mindset, when instead, after actually talking openly with Rachel, found that she didn't want me to have all the answers to 'fix' her. She just wanted me to help make her smile and pick her up on the tough days.

Also understanding what was going wrong inside Rachel's body (which at the time was her T4 medication not converting to enough T3) was an important part of feeling like I could grasp what was happening.

Coping With Mood Swings

Adam's Insights

When I saw changes in Rachel's mood, including mood swings, I had to remind myself that *it wasn't her*. It was her thyroid condition. That it wasn't her choice to feel all these various emotions, sometimes close together. It was something she was working through and trying to understand herself. Instead of getting frustrated or put out by it, or questioning it too much, I learnt to just enjoy the good swings, whilst being aware that a low mood swing may be just around the corner. And after a while, I was even able to identify the warning signs of a low mood swing coming, meaning I could adapt to stop the snowball from getting any bigger.

A lot of coping with your loved one having a mental health condition and coming out of it stronger comes from good communication and paying attention to the build-up.

Watching closely for the cues that certain things might be making things worse, and taking mental notes of what works.

It has involved trial and error and I still get it wrong every now and then, but I know that generally, she prefers to be left alone if she's experiencing mood swings and encouraging her to go for a walk or get outside helps her to feel like she's worked through the swing. Try to pinpoint with your loved one, what does and doesn't help in these moments. Also communicate how you feel when a mood swing strikes.

Chapter 7: How Hypothyroidism Is Going to Change Your Life Too

"It's OK to not have it all figured out yet." - Rachel Hill, The Invisible Hypothyroidism

By Adam

When Rachel was first diagnosed with hypothyroidism, I never thought that her diagnosis would change my life so much. At first, I thought that as long as she stuck to having her medication, life would go back to normal pretty quickly. Having been through the challenges of getting her back on track, and optimal, I have grown to see that this initial thought, whilst well intentioned, is a little naive. Our relationship was bound to change, we had to tackle this as a 'team'.

The biggest difference in our relationship is one of balance. We've had to re-adjust the way we do things, and reset the way we flow with each other. I'm a firm believer that every good long-term relationship gets into a rhythm in order to get through life's struggles together. This could be a rhythm as practical as who takes out the bins or as emotional as who remembers the family and friends birthdays. Both the physical tasks and the non-physical tasks take effort, and some people are better than others at each. For example, Rachel carries the personality trait of a HSP (Highly Sensitive

Person), which means that she is very good at being thoughtful and thinking of other people. This makes her brilliant at finding thoughtful and meaningful presents for things like birthdays or holidays, but she also enjoys keeping a clean and ordered house, something that I can certainly say is not the case for my home office desk. I enjoy gardening, and will quite happily take the heavy lifting associated with keeping our green spaces tidy, or the heavier lifting parts of doing the housework. This flow means that each of us can contribute to the relationship and take advantage of our strengths and this has adjusted the most since Rachel's thyroid disease diagnosis.

After Rachel was diagnosed and going through a really rough patch of her health, this rhythm started to get out of sync. All of a sudden, I had to start considering taking on more responsibility of things that Rachel had always done, or was simply better at. At first, things just gradually stopped getting done, Rachel's brain fog or lack of energy meant that she wasn't able to keep up. She would often hide this to keep the appearance that things were carrying on as "normal" as she didn't want her diagnosis to get in the way of something she took pride in, being thoughtful and keeping a tidy house.

Often when I tried to help, I would get in the way, only causing more tension and generally getting things wrong. It took several conversations and many months for me to understand the type of support that she now needed. She was still the same person inside, one that genuinely wanted to remember peoples' birthdays and keep a tidy, relaxing house, but it was her body and hypothyroidism letting her down and going against her in the ability to do these.

We had to change our rhythm, our flow, in order for us to succeed again as a couple. This meant understanding the things she needed from me, and her understanding a realistic expectation of what I could get done too. This required change. Something that is scary for all of us. This process took time, lots of readjustments, and a continuous dialogue, one that we maintain to this day about the type of support that I can best provide.

With her brain fog and lack of energy, a lot of the responsibility for getting through the day-to-day tasks rested on my shoulders. This meant making decisions for both of us, even when Rachel wasn't able to contribute to the decision-making process. This can seem quite daunting, you're having to wade through a lot of information, choices and decisions, but by taking the time to reflect and look after both of our well-beings, we were able to evade the hardest parts of her recovery, together.

I'm happy to say that now Rachel's hypothyroidism is well managed, things have returned to somewhat of a 'normal'/pre-hypothyroidism balance. Things are still different, I do need to make sure I keep an eye on her ongoing energy levels, or provide a loving comment here and there when I think she's taking on too much.

Try to approach this change with the best of intentions. Getting frustrated, or longing for a time before diagnosis will not help either of you. I know Rachel longed for her health more than I longed for the time we spent before her diagnosis. As a loved one you are exposed to the changes in their lifestyle, but you never have to live them yourself. Trying to keep this in mind and accepting the challenge of being together now in different circumstances can actually make your relationship stronger. We certainly understand each other better now than we ever did before her diagnosis. I wouldn't wish this change on any couple, but it is one where, with time, love and dedication can make you both flourish.

Part Two: Spouses and Romantic Partners

Information for spouses, other halves and partners of those with hypothyroidism.

Chapter 8: What Is It like Living with a Hypothyroid Partner?

"There are golden days and there are dark days. Remember to enjoy things when the sun is shining." - Adam Gask

By Adam

I wrote this after a particularly hard day of trying to support Rachel through her physical and mental health struggles.

Originally written as an online article, I felt it was important to share it in this book to provide validation to what I expect many other partners of those with hypothyroidism experience.

What is it like living with a hypothyroid partner?

Hard. There is no clearer way to say it.

There are good days, bad days and golden days. It's a struggle mentally, physically and emotionally, for both you and for her.

On the bad days, you need to keep going. Just keep on going. Just keep on swimming. To make sure you remember that no matter how tired you are, how mentally drained you feel, how emotionally unstable you may feel, it is nothing compared to how she feels. Nothing. Not even close. Forget it.

You need to step up, carry the extra weight or burdens in order to make things a little easier. Because she needs you. She wants you to be there for her.

On the bad days, it can hit you like a tonne of bricks from nowhere. And over time you need to build up a tolerance to the bad days, to take more in your stride and know how to handle them. To have a cool head and be the mast in the storm you're both going through. It can happen last thing at night, during the night or first thing in the morning. It can be the smallest or it can be the biggest of things. You get better over time at judging what makes things worse or simply doesn't help, but you'll never get it 100% right. Know that and work with that. You just learn to try and not make the same mistakes twice.

As time goes on I've come to know that on those bad days, you can be both the hero and villain all at once. To be the hero they need to make sure they can keep putting one step in front of the other, the villain to make sure they get to bed on time and take those supplements or do the routines she hates.

You come to treasure the things that make her better. Being the one to make her that breakfast which makes her feel better first thing, or to help her have those few more spoons. To make sure she does take the car and not walk, even though she really wants to, because you want to make sure she can get through to lunchtime, where you can go and see her to bring her some chocolate. To be the one who brings that spark back in her, that you both remember.

You try so hard to do the little things to help; to do things around the house. To try and make their life that little bit easier. It isn't always enough though, be prepared for that. It might be the wrong word said here, the wrong thing done there, but do the things you know makes things better. That foot massage she needs to be able to sleep. That hot bath with the bubbles she likes, just right - not too hot though. Do the things you said you'd do. Pick up your socks. Do the washing up. Make that extra trip to the shop when she's feeling low. Get her favourite ice cream. Do the things only you know to make sure she gets everything she needs to feel better.

Because when she does feel better, those are the Golden days. The days where everything feels that little bit normal. The days where you can be the ages you really are. To be with the one you fell in love with all day instead of in glimpses. Those days don't happen all that often. They require the stars to align just right. Sometimes you can get close, and those are the good days. Days where we might be able to do all the things we wanted to do. To be silly. To laugh together. To cuddle and watch all the things we want to. To watch that next episode of F.R.I.E.N.D.S. To get Netflix to ask "Are you still watching". These are the golden days that make it all worth it. And it is all worth it.

Seeing Your Loved One Go from Healthy to Poor Health

Nothing can prepare you for seeing the person you love go from a happy-go-lucky, bubbly and exuberant person to a complete shell. A shadow of their former selves.

We had some really dark times during the worst of Rachel's hypothyroidism journey. I would go to work hoping that whilst she was sick in bed, struggling physically and mentally, that she wouldn't act on feeling suicidal. It was a constant battle of trying to remain positive in front of her, trying to find solutions, being the rock she needed and maintaining a level head. Looking after both her and my mental health wasn't easy.

I was fortunate (in an odd sort of way) that everything was so intense that all I could do was focus on helping her. I didn't have enough time to sit and reflect on where I was in all of this. It was just a constant turn of the wheel each day to try and keep us both above water. A gradual decline, I can assume would allow for more reflection and doubt on whether Hypothyroidism was at the root cause of the major change in Rachel's life. Instead, everything happened really quickly once she started getting major symptoms, which helped point the finger at that small gland in her neck after not too long.

I did have moments where I wished things would return to how they used to be. After she was on the road to recovery, it felt like the issues and complications wouldn't stop. I really did miss the woman I fell in love with. But the thing that kept me going was seeing glimpses of that person still in our day to day.

At first they were fleeting, a laugh I remembered, or a smile, before returning for longer periods of time. A trip out or a visit to somewhere where we were able to be a 'normal' couple. I refer to these moments as 'golden moments', times where the hypothyroidism wasn't actively present in our relationship and we got to just be ourselves.

I came to really appreciate these times, but I never really knew when they would appear. I would try and ensure the likelihood was as high as can be, making sure that things were as clean as possible at home, that work and life were in balance and that I was ensuring she had the attention she needed to know she was loved. These patches of time, have thankfully grown in length and quantity, now more so than ever. But, being close to Rachel for so long and seeing the rollercoaster ride that is hypothyroidism, I know that the 'dark days', the ones that are of complete opposite to the 'golden days' can happen at any time too. These 'dark days' are things that I have had to grow accustomed to and ultimately accept. Rejecting them or hoping that they will not reappear is neither realistic nor helpful. I now approach these with more experience than ever, and a drive to make them as short as possible.

I often still say the wrong thing or do the wrong thing when things are bad, or when the 'dark days' are hanging around for longer than usual. But I do strive to try and learn from these. There are mistakes that I have only learnt by keeping a dialogue open with Rachel after everything has cleared up.

By focusing on reducing the 'bad days' and cherishing the 'golden days', I now no longer wish or grieve for the person I met in 2009. The person before hypothyroidism. But instead see that this disease has made her so much stronger, and only enhanced the best qualities of her, as she has now come to appreciate when things are going well to take full advantage. On a whole, her health is very good most days, but she still goes through flare ups from time to time. They say to live each day as if it's your last, and whilst I don't fully subscribe to that, I do believe in taking full advantage of when the sun is shining.

Chapter 9: Fertility, Pregnancy and Parenting with Hypothyroidism

"The idea of having a child and being responsible for looking after someone else, when some days I can't even look after myself, is scary." - Rachel Hill, The Invisible Hypothyroidism

Many couples are excited at the prospect of starting a family, but for those with hypothyroidism, there can be an added layer of worry *and* complication.

Not only does having hypothyroidism increase the chances of pregnancy complications such as miscarriage, pre-eclampsia, anaemia, stillbirth and the baby developing congenital hypothyroidism itself, but a thyroid patient's health during pregnancy and after birth can also be quite uncertain.

Fertility

In women, thyroid hormones directly affect the uterine lining, which can cause infertility or miscarriages to occur when they are abnormal. As well as complications during pregnancy, some women with low thyroid levels may even struggle to fall pregnant at all.

Infertility can occur when thyroid hormones are low and TRH (thyrotropin-releasing hormone) which is responsible for stimulating the pituitary gland to release prolactin, causes the increased prolactin to interfere with the ovulation process. The increased prolactin levels can prevent the ovaries from releasing an egg each month, which makes it more difficult to conceive.

I am also noticing more and more hypothyroid women

with sex hormone issues such as oestrogen dominance, which can affect cycles and ovulation. Since the thyroid, pituitary and ovaries are all part of the endocrine system, it's not difficult to see why having a problem with one of these, may also mean having issues with another.

In men with hypothyroidism, erectile dysfunction, delayed ejaculation, sperm abnormalities, infertility issues and low testosterone levels are often reported and can affect starting a family too.

However, both males and females with hypothyroidism can improve their fertility chances by ensuring that thyroid levels, TSH, Free T3 and Free T4 (and Reverse T3 if possible) as well as thyroid antibodies, are all optimal. Addressing any oestrogen dominance, low testosterone or other hormonal imbalances, would also be a good place to start. Chapter 2 discusses what we should look for in test results when aiming for 'optimal' treatment.

I wouldn't recommend trying to conceive unless thyroid levels are definitely optimised and the all-clear has been given from a medical professional, as not doing so puts the unborn child at risk of complications, but also the pregnant thyroid patient. I would be concerned about the physical and mental health of both parents involved if they were to go through a complicated pregnancy or pregnancy loss. So, try to avoid this at all costs by getting your ducks in a row first.

Once Pregnant

If your hypothyroid partner is female, then as soon they know they're pregnant, they should inform their doctor and get a full thyroid panel arranged as soon as possible.

In the first part of pregnancy, the foetus relies completely on the mother to provide thyroid hormone for its development. For someone with a perfectly healthy thyroid gland and function, their body is able to meet that extra demand rather easily, but in a woman with hypothyroidism, her body may not be able to.

According to the Endocrine Society's 2007 Clinical Guidelines for the Management of Thyroid Dysfunction during Pregnancy and Postpartum, thyroid medication usually needs to be increased in dosage, by four to six week gestation and may well require a 30-50% increase in dosage. [10]

Most women with hypothyroidism require an increase in thyroid medication when pregnant, to support the developing baby. Failure to properly maintain adequate thyroid levels whilst pregnant can result in complications such as miscarriage, pre-eclampsia, anaemia, stillbirth and congenital hypothyroidism. So, it's very important to be tested regularly, often every four to six weeks throughout pregnancy. Adjustments to medication should then be made accordingly, with the guidance of a medical professional.

It is understood that poor brain development and congenital hypothyroidism can be attributed to poorly managed hypothyroidism during pregnancy, as well as risk of tragically losing the pregnancy. Some researchers believe that one factor in the development of autism is severe hypothyroidism in the mother. So, supporting the thyroid patient in your life by helping them advocate and look after their thyroid health when it comes to pregnancy is very important.

Mental Health and Pregnancy

Postnatal depression could also be due to low thyroid function and this is important to be aware of. If your partner has been told that they have postnatal or antenatal depression, then it is definitely worth them having a full thyroid panel conducted to check thyroid function. In fact, I feel that thyroid screening should become mandatory during and after all pregnancies.

Postnatal and antenatal depression are real mental health conditions in their own right, but for someone with an existing thyroid condition, it would be irresponsible to disregard it as a possible reason for poor mental health during or after a pregnancy.

During Pregnancy and Post-Pregnancy

Predicting what a thyroid patient's health is going to be like during pregnancy and after giving birth is nigh on impossible, but it doesn't mean you can't be prepared. Whereas some women with hypothyroidism report feeling better when pregnant, for many others, they feel worse and this can get worse following delivering their baby too, due to thyroid hormone levels needing time to settle back in to place post-birth.

You can prepare for needing more support than the average couple by building a support network prior to the baby's arrival, such as people you can count on to help cook meals, do laundry or otherwise help you out.

Thyroid hormone levels can take anywhere from a few weeks to a few months to iron out in women with hypothyroidism who have given birth, and this should be taken into consideration too. For some women, they may also benefit from seeing a functional medicine practitioner, naturopath or other progressive medicine practitioner, for addressing of adrenal health, stress and holistic support following a birth.

Maximising how much time they get to sleep, rest and recuperate will go a long way in getting her health back on track so she can be as conscious and present a parent as possible.

Adam's Insights

The biggest thing I want to stress for this topic is the concept of being prepared. If you can make sure that you are both as clued up as possible and as involved as you can be, it will really help when you go through the life changing event of becoming parents.

Thyroid symptoms such as brain fog, fatigue and mood swings can increase during pregnancy, so it's useful to ensure that you, the non-thyroid patient, are present to ask questions and be an extra pair of ears to listen and remember key information (for example at medical appointments or prenatal classes). It may be that your hypothyroid partner also feels more easily overwhelmed during pregnancy, so ensuring you are in this together will help you both.

The chances are that her thyroid levels will go up and down throughout pregnancy and this may mean that she swings between better health and worse health days. So, if you're able to take notes at appointments, in prenatal classes and be proactive, it will help.

It is also worth bearing in mind that in this situation, you're supporting everyone involved; your hypothyroid partner and unborn child. It can be quite a scary concept but, by being clued up, you can avoid various issues with the pregnancy, birth and post-birth.

Raising Children When You're Hypothyroid

Raising a family when you have hypothyroidism can understandably also bring with it added things to juggle. Just like during pregnancy, predicting someone's thyroid health when they have the added task of everything that comes with parenthood can become tricky. We all have an idea of who we want to be as parents, so imagine the guilt, regret and feelings of failure your loved one may feel when they feel as if they're coming up short due to their health condition leaving them with less energy, less time and less of the stuff they want to do in order to be a 'perfect parent'. Of course, you probably feel that they are in fact doing enough, but they may not be feeling that way themselves.

As you've probably gathered by now, thyroid patients are often known to push themselves each and every day to keep on going, keep on raising their families with love and kindness despite their own body fighting against them. Many parents with hypothyroidism are even more exhausted, even more stressed and struggle even more so mentally, as well as physically, than other parents. On thyroid flare up days, pulling the laundry out of the washing machine can be exhausting, showering can use up all their energy and cooking the family a nutritious meal might not be an option if they're so fatigued and in pain that they're struggling to stand for long.

It's hard to say for any of us, whether our health will A) bounce back after beginning parenthood B) take a while and a mixture of different health practitioners to iron it back out or C) never truly be the same. However, if you already have children, you probably know better than anyone else how it affects your loved one, as you witness them trying to maintain this balance as best they can every day. If you embark on the journey of raising a family together, it may be that at times you need to remind them to check in with their doctor to have their thyroid levels checked and medication reviewed, as juggling their own medications, medical appointments and check-ups for themselves, let alone all the ones for your child or children too, can become overwhelming. And there's a good chance they'll be putting the kids first almost all the time.

When you have children, being realistic about both of your responsibilities as parents, such as whether you need to pull in help from a wider circle of support, is crucial. Those extended family members and close friends can help to pick up the slack when a parent's hypothyroidism flares. For example, if your hypothyroid partner can't play sports with your child right now, you may have a friend who can play sports with them during this flare.

Talking to children about their parent's health condition can seem tricky and there's no right or wrong way to handle it really, but often being honest and keeping them in the loop with when their parent is having a rest day can be useful in helping them understand. On these more difficult days, they may be able to help out with making the dinner (even if it's just washing the vegetables), setting the table or carrying a load of laundry to the washing machine. They may even value the importance of eating healthily if they understand why their hypothyroid parent follows certain dietary advice for managing their thyroid condition. Saying this, it is also important to not put too much responsibility on children when harder health times strike, so remembering to pull in help from fellow surrounding adults is important too.

It might be that if you have a family, depending on your own personal situation, that your finances take a bit of a hit if the hypothyroid parent becomes a stay at home parent. Of course, many people around the world become stay at home parents without a health condition, but for those with an existing health condition, they may find that in order to get the balance right between being a parent with a chronic illness and juggling everything else life has to offer, that they give up work for some time and this can of course affect your finances. Especially as children are not cheap! Many couples struggle with conversations surrounding the topic of money, so be sure to be realistic and honest in how this may change for you both and how you'll manage this change. A financial planner may be extra useful here.

Having a chronic illness such as hypothyroidism may even change your plans about having children or, after having one child, having more. It's possible that a pregnancy with hypothyroidism can be a bit of an ordeal, or perhaps the pregnancy wasn't particularly eventful but parenthood has your other half experiencing more bad thyroid days than manageable ones. Again, whether you discuss keeping your family small or whether options that negate the need for pregnancy, such as adoption, are an option, these are all important conversations to have when the time comes.

Support groups for parents in the community can be a lifeline. Regular meetups at parks, libraries, and more can provide great friendship, reassurance and support to both mothers and fathers. It may be that you utilise this form of support too, as it is possible that you may be able to connect with other parents that have a chronically ill other half.

Chapter 10: Libido and Sex

"Sex is as important as eating or drinking." - *Marquis de Sade*

The loss of libido (sex drive) when someone has hypothyroidism is very common. Thyroid hormones are needed for regulating metabolism, heart rate, temperature, blood pressure and they can even affect libido.

The thyroid hormone T3 just so happens to be vital in the functioning of both the ovaries and testes, whereby too little available T3 can cause the sex drive to go out of business and diminish. Remember how we said thyroid hormones are needed for every function and every cell? Yes, even sexual functions and arousal.

We also know that low thyroid hormones can also cause people to feel low in mood, irritable, overly-emotional, fatigued and achy. Would you always want to have sex when you feel so unwell and rubbish? For many, the changes to their sex drives and sex life can be down to a mixture of low thyroid hormone levels but also feeling rubbish physically and mentally.

Adams Insights

After speaking to Rachel at length about this topic, I've found that the best way to understand her point of view is like this:

Imagine someone has cooked you your favourite meal. It has everything you could possibly imagine. It's perfect; the best sirloin steak, the best thin crust pizza, your

89

favourite curry. It's got everything, every possible accompaniment, every side order and your favourite drink to wash it all down with. Except, you're not hungry because you feel sick. You'd love to demolish the entire thing, but can't. It doesn't appeal to you at all. No matter how much you'd like to eat it, you have no appetite and feel so ill. That is what having a low libido with hypothyroidism can feel like. It's not a case of desire, it's a case of situation. When a chronic illness can make you feel ill every day, sex may not be the top of your priorities.

As well as thyroid hormones, adrenal hormones can also become involved. Many people with hypothyroidism also find they have adrenal fatigue (note: it is more accurately referred to as hypothalamic-pituitary axis dysfunction), a separate condition that is identified by having too much or too little of the stress hormone cortisol. However, the adrenals are also involved in the synthesis of DHEA, testosterone, aldosterone, oestrogen and progesterone, other important hormones. All are especially important to your libido. All of these share the same precursor, pregnenolone.

The link between your libido and adrenals occurs here. When adrenal fatigue exists in the form of high cortisol, it can start to 'steal' more progesterone than is ideal, as it's a building block for cortisol, in order to produce more cortisol and maintain high levels. This can lead to oestrogen dominance, where the ratio of oestrogen to progesterone is unbalanced. Imbalances in these hormones can affect our sex drive, ability to become aroused, interest in sex and even vaginal dryness and how comfortable we feel during sex. In men with hypothyroidism, erectile dysfunction, fertility issues, low testosterone levels, slow facial hair growth, premature balding or thinning of hair and reduced muscle mass can also indicate hormonal imbalances.

As well as the thyroid patient in your life ensuring that they are optimally treated for their thyroid condition, they can also address any other hormonal imbalances to restore their libido and as a loved one, you will need to remain understanding and patient with their situation.

I understand that it can be difficult when you're in a relationship and perhaps only one half wants to have that level of intimacy right now, but honestly, when someone is chronically ill, emotionally, mentally and physically drained, it just may not be a priority in comparison to other parts of the day. They may be just too tired to even think about sex. Even undressing can feel like too much effort when your libido and energy are zapped. Yes, it can strain the relationship, but whilst sexual intimacy is an important part of many loving relationships and marriages, it forms one piece of a much bigger puzzle.

I can understand the stress of someone who wants to show their partner how much they mean to them sexually, but having their partner uninterested. I understand the concern this causes and the worry it generates. It's only natural! But you need to talk and remain open and honest about all of this, from both sides. If your sex life has been affected whilst the thyroid patient in your life is coming to terms with their thyroid condition and getting it under control, I assure you that it is no one's fault, but it is down to both of you to work through it.

The good news is, that when low thyroid hormone levels are corrected, as well as sex hormone levels and adrenal dysfunction if applicable, the result is often a return to all bodily functions and processes, including the libido.

Adam's Insights

Knowing that hypothyroidism or adrenal issues can affect libido is really important. Like many cis men, I'm pretty much always 'in the mood' for sexual intimacy, and it can be difficult to grasp that your partner may not be. Especially if their sex drive used to be much higher. But try to remember that they haven't chosen for this to happen, so try to avoid making comparisons between how they were a few years ago and how they are now. Life is always changing and that's just life - but talking to your partner about how you feel can help. They often recognise this absence in your relationship too and may feel guilty, but opening up and talking ensures that you can clear the air between you.

When the body is struggling, as it often is with hypothyroidism, it makes sense that sex may be the last thing on your partner's mind. This is often hard to come to terms with.

With hypothyroidism also having the tendency to change a person's appearance, whether that be weight changes, skin changes (acne and eczema for example), hair loss etc. do also remind your significant other that you still love them and find them attractive. It's not uncommon for their confidence to be knocked when physical changes that they can't control occur. It's possible they might even think you don't find them as attractive. A lack of confidence can also contribute to not wanting to be sexually intimate.

You can also be intimate together in other ways than sex. Back massages, walks without mobile phones and instead concentrating on talking to each other, date nights, making a point of reserving days/evenings just for you two - these can all make you feel closer and often build intimacy in the way that it can naturally lead on to more of a desire to be sexually intimate together. Reconnect with each other, doing the things you often did before hypothyroidism and try to avoid getting frustrated about it - this won't help the situation. What can help is focusing on what you can do now. You'll find your way back to regular sexual intimacy with a strengthened connection.

Part Three: Friends, Family and Those That Live with a Thyroid Patient

Information for the friends, family and those who live with someone that has hypothyroidism.

Chapter 11: Having a Child with Hypothyroidism

"Any parent who says parenting came easily to them is not being honest with themselves. Parenting is hard." - Karamo Brown

Having a child with a health condition can certainly be worrying. As with all health conditions, catching and diagnosing hypothyroidism early on can greatly help to prevent or minimise the possible effects on the child's life and development.

Children and teenagers who develop hypothyroidism typically have the same signs and symptoms as adults do (which are listed in Chapter 2), but they may also experience poor growth, develop their adult teeth later than other children, have delayed puberty and poor mental development.

However, for those *born* with hypothyroidism (called congenital hypothyroidism), they can look 'normal' and have no obvious symptoms, which is why it is so important that all children be tested at birth or soon after.

Children That Develop Hypothyroidism

Children and teenagers that develop hypothyroidism usually have a family history of the disease. Parents may notice a change in their energy levels, concentration, mood and physical appearance. Weight gain despite no real change in their diet or exercise routine could indicate hypothyroidism, as well as a lack of appetite or energy to exercise as much as they used to.

Children with undiagnosed hypothyroidism may appear to be 'behind' their peers in several ways, such as in height, mental development and missing school due to frequent illness. Female teenagers may experience period problems such as a delayed start to commencing their menstrual cycles, heavy, absent or irregular periods, possibly even accompanied by migraines.

A full thyroid panel (consisting of TSH, Free T3, Free T4, Thyroid Peroxidase Antibodies, Thyroglobulin Antibodies and Reverse T3 if possible too) can give the most comprehensive overview of thyroid health, including diagnosing if a child or teenager has hypothyroidism. However, as hypothyroidism is most often diagnosed in middle aged women, many doctors may not think to check children with symptoms for thyroid disease, so you may need to really insist that levels are checked. Signs that their medication may not be optimally treating their thyroid condition can include any of the symptoms listed in Chapter 2, or mentioned in this chapter.

Treatment for children or teenagers with hypothyroidism is the same as adults, where medication is usually needed for life. The medication type given is most often T4-only, such as Levothyroxine or Synthroid, which seems to work well for most, though may prove less beneficial as the child ages and after a certain age it may be worth considering a T3 and T4 combination. Full thyroid panel testing is usually carried out once a year or (more preferably) once every six months once levels are stabilised. You may be worried about your child handling all the appointments, blood draws and medication. There's no easy way to manage this and all children are of course different, but there may well be some tears. One of the biggest parts to your child having a positive blood draw experience is in how you handle the event. Try to remain relaxed – children can easily pick up on your emotions and assume that if you're worried about it, they should be too. Planning a treat or something fun for afterwards can help.

Remember that often you will be your child's health advocate until they reach an age where they naturally take it on themselves. If you feel that they're not receiving the best care, you are entitled to speak up, ask questions and find another healthcare practitioner if you wish.

Congenital Hypothyroidism

The term 'congenital' means that a condition is present at birth. Congenital hypothyroidism is therefore present in an infant from birth and it is usually diagnosed at birth, too. Screening is performed at about five days old, with a heel-prick blood test.

Congenital hypothyroidism can be hereditary and the most common cause of hypothyroidism in children is a family history of the disease. For some babies with congenital hypothyroidism, their thyroid gland does not form in its normal position in the neck, in others, the gland does not develop at all and for others, it is underdeveloped.

The National Academy of Hypothyroidism estimates that 1 in every 2000-4,000 children in the US are born with hypothyroidism[11]. That's about 3000 a year in the UK according to the BTF[12].

Some babies with hypothyroidism are sleepy and difficult to feed, although lots of babies have these symptoms without being hypothyroid. Other symptoms in babies with congenital hypothyroidism may include constipation, a high birth weight, low muscle tone, dry skin, low body temperature and poor growth. As long as it is caught early on and medicated correctly, it should not greatly impact the child's life.

However, if standard T4-only medication (such as Synthroid and Levothyroxine) doesn't seem to be helping their symptoms as they age, do know that there are other medication options, such as synthetic T3 which can be taken alone or added to synthetic T4, as well as NDT preparations and compounded medication, both of which contain all five thyroid hormones. Some doctors may be hesitant to try these less conventional medication options on children, but it may be worth the discussion.

Being told that your newborn child has a lifelong condition, for which they will need to take medication daily for the rest of their lives, can be hugely overwhelming. Mothers may even look to blame themselves for missing it or look for reasons why it may have happened but the important thing to remember is that it can be managed and you will settle in to this new normal.

Chapter 12: Seeing Your Friend or Family Member Struggle

"So many people love and appreciate you. Don't focus on the ones that don't." - Rachel Hill, The Invisible Hypothyroidism

Seeing a friend or family member that was formerly active, bright eyed, switched-on and lively, go through the diagnosis of hypothyroidism and perhaps become less active, more fatigued, brain fogged and not as happy, can be incredibly hard. There is likely *so much* that you want to do for them but feel as if you have no idea how to help.

Living with hypothyroidism can take over lives. Whereas some people with it feel better rather quickly with thyroid medication, others can take months or even years to start feeling better. The path back to better health is very much individual.

However, for many, it changes their lives forever. Whether in many major ways or a few, small ways.

So, to those of you who have a friend or family member with hypothyroidism, I imagine it can be frustrating having your once very reliable and sociable friend, now perhaps not-so reliable, not-so available or not-so sociable.

As you read this chapter, I ask that you remember that the person you know with hypothyroidism did not ask for this disease, and they are just as frustrated as you are, that it can affect their life so much.

Here are four main things you should keep in mind:

1. They Don't like Cancelling on You

Living with thyroid disease can be unpredictable. The thyroid patient in your life may feel well one day and then be struck down the next with a flare up (an increase in thyroid symptoms such as heavy fatigue, muscle aches and pains and brain fog, as explained in Chapter 4). They may feel quite well when they first agree to certain plans with you, and then a few days before, or on the day itself, become really unwell. In fact, going could make them worse.

Many people with hypothyroidism experience flu-like symptoms, and really do try their best to juggle life whilst having a chronic illness. Yet, can be disheartened by needing time to recuperate or look after their health. Please try to understand and in fact, encourage us to rest when you can see that we ought to.

People may think we're lazy or just not making the effort when we have to cancel plans, but when this is our life, we have no real control over how we feel on that particular day.

If we cancel plans unannounced, it doesn't mean we don't want to see you. Talk to us and we'll arrange another time to catch up!

2. Turning up Unannounced Isn't a Fun Surprise and Neither Are Last Minute Plans

It might seem odd that, given my explanation of how we may even need to cancel on long standing plans above, that last minute plans aren't really useful either.

In order to prepare for a social event, meeting or a quick catch up, it can take us days or even weeks of preparation. We may be resting as much as we can before the day so that we're able to make it as much as possible, but we also often need to plan rest days afterwards to recuperate. Social situations can be draining for us in every single way – emotionally, mentally and physically.

So, turning up on our doorstep out the blue, when we haven't had the chance to prepare, muster up the energy to wash and get dressed or tidy the house, can be anxiety-inducing.

And asking us on Saturday morning if we want to meet for lunch that day likely isn't great either. Again, we may need to prep before.

3. We Can Have up and down Days/ Weeks/Months

As I explained in detail in Chapter 4, Hypothyroidism can come with flare ups. Sometimes we know the triggers, so we avoid them and are able to limit flare ups to some extent. But we don't always know what causes them, or we have a 'crash', where we've done too much recently and come to a complete halt, practically sofa-bound.

This means that whilst I was well enough to go to a gig last week, as well as a night out with friends, or I've had a month of being really sociable, it doesn't automatically mean I'm well enough this week or this month, like a regular, healthy person.

You have to treat each day individually where living with thyroid disease is concerned, so don't think we're being rude if we turn down your invite so we can rest up, even though you saw we were 'well enough' to be out earlier in the week. We have to schedule in rest days or we'll make ourselves even more ill. We may not be able to make every event we're invited to so have to figure out which ones we can.

Adam's Insights

I think it's important to understand that the thyroid patient in your life may not be able to keep up with things as well as you can (a healthier person, for example). You may find that you're able to socialise as much as you really want to and that socialising doesn't drain you or have other detrimental effects - but this isn't the case with my hypothyroid spouse.

I've seen how worn out Rachel can get if we schedule too many social events on workday evenings, or fill up weekends with social commitments too. I personally feed off social events and find I have more energy both during and afterwards. But Rachel is the opposite, and her pace for these events is very much different to mine. It might take some trial and error but talking to each other about what works for both of you can help you plan and manage your time effectively.

4. We Really Do Appreciate Thoughtful Gestures

Asking us how we are, suggesting we schedule in a phone call catch-up, sending a card or a little something in the post, can really remind us that there are people who do care, when we feel so rubbish and controlled by our health conditions.

As thyroid patients, we may feel like a burden sometimes, or disregarded by friends we don't get to see as much. Sending things in the post is something I don't think we do enough of these days, as it's becoming much less common. But receiving a mystery card, letter or parcel is somewhat magical and knowing someone has thought of you is heart-warming. It's a simple gesture, but says a lot. I have an article on my website for care package ideas that go down well with hypothyroid patients.

Other thoughtful gestures can include just taking the time to check that we're OK with a text or phone call. We have a tendency to clam up and not disclose everything we're going through, but being able to speak about it to someone every once in a while is a healthy release.

Chapter 13: Why 'How Are You?' Is Such a Difficult Question to Answer

"Be a rainbow in someone else's cloud." - Maya Angelou

"How are you?" is a question that demonstrates someone cares, yet it can be tricky to answer as a thyroid patient. I never really know how to answer it.

It's a question I dread. If I'm asked in person, I sometimes smile and say, "Yeah, I'm fine," and other times I just shrug my shoulders, not wanting to answer, but also not knowing what to say, if I'm honest!

When someone sends me a text asking me how I am and I don't know how to respond, I may leave it unread until I have an answer formed and ready to reply with, but I dread responding. *What if they prod for more information? After all, they're only trying to be caring and thoughtful.*

Many people living with health conditions that affect them day to day, can struggle to answer this question, but I'm not here to tell you to stop asking it or to stop caring. Please don't, we love that you care!

But how do we answer that question when we can't make sense of how we're feeling ourselves? As a thyroid patient, I worry that if I always say I'm not doing too great, it desensitises what I'm going through and people will think I'm being overdramatic.

So, some days it is just easier to say I'm fine and nod. Other days I can't bring myself to lie because I don't have the physical or mental energy to. I might say I'm struggling, in pain or that I don't know how to answer it, and people tend to respond with, "I hope you feel better soon." Again, it's supposed to be a nice and reassuring comment, but I feel more upset knowing that I won't be all better soon. Because I have this condition for the rest of my life.

Your loved one with thyroid disease may not know whether to be honest with you or to "put on a brave face" when you ask them how they're doing. They may want to tell you that every inch of their body is tired and they don't really know why. But they also don't want to scare you or push you away.

However, do know that we appreciate you caring enough to ask, so we truly are sorry if we don't know how to reply to, what should be, a sympathetic and simple enough question. But we appreciate that you're thinking about us!

Chapter 14: Housework and Hypothyroidism

"Before hypothyroidism, I never thought there would come a day when I would miss doing the housework." - Rachel Hill, The Invisible Hypothyroidism

I have always been a tidy and organised person. I keep an up to date diary of Adam and I's plans, meetings and reminders and, for the most part, my life is as organised as it can be. This is also reflected in my home and again, always has been.

I've always been happy in a clean and tidy environment and I take pride and comfort in such an environment.

Before becoming sick, I had seemingly endless amounts of energy to do a lot of housework and keep on top of it all without a problem. I moved throughout the house, cleaning and dancing to my music and enjoying the process. I was pretty particular when it came to cleanliness and how I liked my home environment to be.

But when hypothyroidism struck, it changed this thyroid patient's ability to keep on top of it!

When at my worst with thyroid disease, I could go weeks between getting any housework done. Some weeks, all I could manage was ten minutes at most and it still wiped me out for the rest of the day. Or all I could manage was putting one load of laundry into the washing machine before needing to rest again.

Adam noticed when I became less able and began to try and help out more around the house.

I'd had the ability to take pride in my home and keep it in a way that kept my stress and anxiety levels low taken away.

It made me feel inadequate and, at times, pathetic. It made me feel out of control. It made me feel like the hypothyroidism was yet again winning. It made me feel like I no longer had a defining role in my own household.

It can be tough when a condition we're told is easy to treat can affect our lives in every possible way. From work, to social and love life and even keeping on top of the ironing.

Being able to help out the thyroid patient you know who may be struggling with this part of their lives, can be very much appreciated. Some may feel embarrassed to admit to needing help with it and others may deny it altogether. But even if you can help by washing up the odd glass or plate or loading the washing machine, I'm sure it won't go unappreciated.

Grocery shopping can be just as hard. These days, Adam tends to go on his own and I stay at home using the time to tidy up the house instead. I find grocery shopping is so tiring for me that it's not a good use of my energy.

It is also worth keeping in mind that those who struggle to keep up with housework likely don't appreciate surprise visits from people, as mentioned in Chapter 13. It can be anxiety-inducing for someone to turn up unannounced without being able to prepare yourself. And especially so if you haven't been able to keep on top of housework recently. I would always check that it is OK to visit before you do and give a realistic time of arrival.

Chapter 15: Social Events with Hypothyroidism

"I often find myself weighing up whether a social event is worth the recovery time."- Rachel Hill, The Invisible Hypothyroidism

Many thyroid patients tell me that they wish their friends and family knew how difficult social events can be after developing hypothyroidism.

Social events and activities are great for everyone. Spending time with friends, family or even meeting new people, is said to be good for our mental health and socialising often helps to promote a good work-life balance for those of us who work. However, it can take extra energy for many hypothyroid patients to socialise and recuperate from socialising. Social events can be draining in several ways and can leave us with a 'hangover' effect.

For those of you whose hypothyroid friend or family member was once the life and soul of the party, a social butterfly who loved meeting new people or someone that had a busy social life pre-diagnosis, you may even have witnessed a change in their personality.

Mental Effects

Mentally, those with hypothyroidism can feel exhausted from trying to maintain enthusiasm for discussions and even the ability to follow a lot of stories and updates from several different people. This can be attributed to how hypothyroidism affects how the brain functions.

Thyroid hormone is required for brain function and

111

when thyroid hormone is low, we can seem forgetful, withdrawn, confused and strained. Focusing on making sure we pay as much attention as possible, when we have thyroid brain fog (which can block concentration and the ability to process information) is very mentally draining.

After a social event, we may get home and need to sit in silence for a good while, whilst our mind is still buzzing and trying to process the day! This can have a knock-on effect where we feel physically tired, achy or withdrawn and so we may also need a day or two to recuperate afterwards. It's like being overstimulated. Even loud noises or a disruptive party at the next table in a restaurant can worsen our hypothyroid symptoms and drain us even more.

Physical Effects

People living with a chronic illness, such as hypothyroidism, are often known as 'Spoonies', meaning we can have a limited amount of energy compared to others, and need to plan our energy usage wisely so as to make it through the day. This can result in a simple shower, getting dressed or even brushing our hair becoming exhausting, so before we even arrive to meet you at a social event, we could already be exhausted! (See Chapter 4 for more information on managing energy levels.)

Having to stand at an event can be draining, too, let alone if we're walking from bar to bar or doing some other form of physical activity. Drinking can also worsen hypothyroid symptoms in many people.

Attending a social event in an unfamiliar place, can also be tiring for a few reasons. If applicable, the anxiety and worry we feel over an unusual environment (anxiety seems common with hypothyroid patients) is tiring and can be overwhelming.

It can be concerning to be in an environment where, if we suddenly feel really ill, we have nowhere to escape to, or we feel unsure if they cater to our dietary needs (as many hypothyroidism patients follow gluten-free diets, AIP, Paleo, Keto etc. to help with symptoms). We may have also had to travel or walk a certain distance to reach the location of the event, which uses up more of our limited energy.

If the event is at our house, we've got the hosting to worry about, such as cleaning the house beforehand, ensuring we have all the groceries, preparing and generally being the host, looking after guests and their needs. There is also the cleaning up after an event. For the average person this might be a bit draining or stressful, but it can soon wear someone with a health condition down. Offering to help with any of this will of course be hugely appreciated.

As you can see, thyroid patients can easily become depleted; emotionally, mentally and of course physically. Many have to plan a day or two to recuperate following a social event. Many find themselves weighing up whether a certain social event or situation is worth the recovery time afterwards or if they can afford to spend days recuperating at all, possibly even having to take time off work.

Supporting Them

Through all of this though, it's important to state that many people living with hypothyroidism still like to have an active social life and will try to maintain one wherever possible, but you'll benefit from knowing just how it can affect them.

If they need to head home early or come out a little later in the day, please try to be understanding, and if they're avoiding certain food or even alcohol because of it worsening their health, help them to keep on track with this too. As someone who follows a gluten-free diet myself, I can vouch for it becoming easier to find places with gluten-free menus these days and it's honestly so appreciated when my friends support me in this by looking at online menus with me or trying out new places.

Chapter 16: Understanding and Supporting Dietary Changes

"Everything we put into our bodies has the potential to either help or hinder our health." - Rachel Hill, The Invisible Hypothyroidism

Many people with hypothyroidism, especially the autoimmune kind, are making dietary changes to manage their condition and are seeing great effects. As a thyroid patient who has gone gluten-free, it has helped me to slow down the progression of my autoimmune thyroid disease greatly.[13]

For others, they see the benefits of also going dairy-free, free of soy, grains, all processed food and more. There are many combinations and as already mentioned throughout this book, every person is unique and individual and what helps them can be just as individual too.

However, what they all have in common is the ability to flare up our conditions and make us unwell if we *do* consume them. And this is where your support comes in. Understanding any dietary adjustments we may have made is crucial if we eat with you, around your house or perhaps even receive food from you as gifts.

As an example, if I consume gluten, which creates a flare up in my condition, Adam and I refer to it as being 'glutened'. I've become 'glutened' when served food at a restaurant I was told did not contain gluten, but evidently did when I had to rush to the toilet with stomach cramps, followed by brain fog, and intense hypothyroidism symptoms over the resulting days.

I'm not trying to be awkward and I've never been a fussy

eater, but I have chosen to follow this diet for the sake of my health and well-being. Each time I consume gluten it worsens my condition and encourages more thyroid function to be lost. I know I feel better avoiding gluten, as my condition stays stable and I am able to function more like a regular human being.

When it comes to your own friend or family member who may be following a specific diet or avoiding certain foods, you can be supportive by asking them what ingredients they are looking for on packaging or menus and learning to spot them too.

I wrote a list of all offending forms of gluten for family members and they used this whenever buying or making food for me, until they became confident in knowing exactly what to look for without needing the list. Investing in some cookbooks that cater to your loved one's dietary needs can make cooking for them a whole lot easier and can even be a bonding experience. If they're gluten-free, then gluten-free baking can be quite the adventure! I contributed to Emily Kyle's *The 30-Minute Thyroid Cookbook: 125 Healing Recipes for Hypothyroidism and Hashimoto's* which is the main cookbook we use at home for evening meals.

Helping us protect our health benefits not only the thyroid patient, but those around us too, as we can spend more time enjoying life with you and less time being unwell!

If you share a home with someone who has dietary restrictions such as being gluten-free, then it's worth keeping in mind cross-contamination rules. Separate cooking equipment will be needed, e.g. separate toasters for bread and separate utensils such as wooden spoons, which can hold on to gluten, are necessary.

In our house, we have two toasters, and we mark the

wooden spoons, to show which have been used in gluten-containing foods and which are safe and free of gluten. When we're making dinner, we have to be careful not to mix up things, like for instance, gluten-free pasta and the regular pasta. Work surfaces are cleaned regularly and thoroughly, too, making sure not to contaminate sponges that are used for both of us.

Adam's Insights

In my experience, it can be hard for friends and family to truly understand this part of a thyroid disease diagnosis. Rachel's good friend and my cousin, Liz, is a great example of someone embracing this.

Liz is now as well versed at spotting gluten as Rachel is, even after being gluten-free for years now. Checking all packets, boxes and knowing the list of things Rachel can't eat, we often chuckle at how good Liz is with it, but it really is amazing to see her so committed to understanding Rachel's dietary restrictions. She especially gets excited when she finds something new that Rachel can eat and they can share together.

With Liz being so defensive about protecting Rachel's health in this way, it helps Rachel feel less awkward about her dietary restrictions. She has someone who 'gets it' and makes it a lot less stressful than it could be. Having this kind of person around you is invaluable.

Chapter 17: Difficulties with Working

"My skills include reading a whole email without absorbing a single word."- Rachel Hill, The Invisible Hypothyroidism

A part of being hypothyroid that is often overlooked is the way that it can affect work lives. Whilst for some thyroid patients, they go about living an almost normal life, for many others, remaining in employment can be very challenging.

I was diagnosed with autoimmune hypothyroidism at twenty-one years old and the workplace I was in at the time was luckily very supportive. Though I appreciate that this isn't the same for everyone. My line manager and work colleagues witnessed me going through quite a tough time with testing, increasing symptoms and countless doctor's appointments, until the eventual diagnosis. By this time, I had been at that particular place of work for two years and they had seen my decline and how I struggled to keep up with work like I used to.

For me, my thyroid disease affecting work presented in a reduced ability to make it into the office every day, with most weeks consisting of at least one missed day of work. At one point, I was practically bed-bound due to my poor physical health, with flu-like symptoms and indescribable fatigue weighing my body down.

Other days, it was my mental health - anxiety and depression - also caused by my thyroid condition. A sudden rush of panic as if something awful was going to happen but not being able to pinpoint what exactly, wasn't a rare occurrence. Panic attacks through the night. Night terrors. Not being able to stop crying whilst trying to get ready for work. I was a mental and emotional mess. My life was falling apart and so was I, thanks to thyroid disease.

I was trying to deal with my newly diagnosed lifelong thyroid condition the best I could behind closed doors as I felt too embarrassed to tell any friends or family about it, but it started spilling out into every corner of my life and I couldn't contain the effects of hypothyroidism on my life any longer. I was a wreck and a shell of my former self, and at only twenty-one years old, I thought *'this isn't normal'*.

I'm lucky that people in my workplace were so understanding at the time, as I really struggled to remain in work. But I am well aware this isn't always the case for everyone. As knowledge about hypothyroidism among the general public is so poor, workplaces often aren't aware of how much thyroid disease can cripple people. Doctors refusing to listen about how our hypothyroidism is affecting us and our work lives, are also causing a lot of harm, since this reiterates what our work colleagues and bosses may already think.

This is what a typical workday was like for me before I got my thyroid condition properly addressed:

I go to bed at 8pm because I'm so unbelievably tired. I sleep pretty much straight through the night, maybe waking briefly during the night, but nothing to hugely disturb the amount of sleep I get, before my alarm goes off at 7am for work. That's 11 hours of sleep. Yet I feel more tired than when I went to bed the night before. How is that possible?

I drag myself out of bed, forcing myself to have a shower, get dressed and make my way downstairs. All of this is hard because it's like I'm moving a dead weight. Putting on my trousers left me breathless and getting in the shower almost made me collapse. I'm also a bit dizzy, light headed and weak whilst doing these things, but I manage them, just.

As I make my way out of the house, my legs are trying their best to stop me. Walking to work is draining every ounce of energy I do happen to have left after that shambles of a night's sleep. I feel sick, my heart is pounding and I'm having hot flushes. I'm scared I'm going to pass out but I keep going. I get to work, and even though I have a sedentary office job, it's going to be a longgg day. The room feels freezing, even though everyone in the office doesn't feel the same. When someone opens a window or puts on a fan, my bones ache even more and it makes all my symptoms ten times worse. I struggle to get out of my chair and walk to the toilet. I struggle to get myself a drink or some food, if I even have an appetite for it. I struggle to type on my computer because my fingers individually hurt and my hands are weak.

When the phone rings, my heart jumps with the shock of a loud noise. My reflexes are poor, and my arms are absolutely aching, with this heaviness that's like having weights tied to them, but I manage to answer the phone. I forget for a second what I'm supposed to say, then muster up a "Hello, Rachel speaking. How can I help you?" It comes out quiet and croaky. I feel drained already and it's only 9am. I'm exhausted in every inch of my body. My fingers are heavy and stiff.

For the rest of the day, it's a struggle to get anything done. I can't think straight, and even the simplest of tasks take 100 times more energy than if I weren't so fatigued. I answer the phone again later *and completely forget what I'm supposed to say. I type an email and completely forget halfway through what I was going to type. Someone asked me if I wanted a cup of tea, and I can't compute what they've asked me. I have this mental block.*

Mid-afternoon, I get a sudden slump where I feel even worse. My eyes are now heavier than ever, my blood pressure speeds up and things like back ache and headaches set in. They'll stay with me all day now.

After what feels like a twenty-hour day, I make my way home, barely even standing anymore. My body is punishing me without any reason. Yesterday was a normal day. I didn't overexert myself and I haven't done anything to deserve this struggle today. I get through the front door and collapse on the sofa, just a few feet away from the door. I sleep for a couple hours, before waking up and seeing it's about 8pm, so I make my way to bed, and sleep for another 10-11 hours, maybe even more. If I'm lucky, I might manage to get some food and drink. The fatigue can often make me feel sick, though.

I might sleep through the night, or tonight, despite feeling like I've ran a marathon, I toss and turn and can't get to sleep, knowing how awful I'm going to feel the next morning. I'm in despair and can't bare the next day.

My alarm goes off at 7am for work. I get up feeling more tired than when I went to bed the night before.

The same day unfolds.

* * *

Being suicidally depressed at the time added another layer to my struggle at work too. I had zero motivation and couldn't concentrate on anything. All I could think about was how much physical and mental pain I was in, how drained I was all the time, how totally fed up I was, and basically, how I wanted it to end.

Whether your loved one discloses their health conditions, mental and/or physical, to their employer is up to them. I personally find it much easier, when starting any new job, to disclose quite early on that I live with X, Y and Z, and "this is how they can affect me". Often, the perfect example will present itself for this, such as a doctor's appointment during work hours, opening the conversation between me and my employer.

I like to make my line manager and work colleagues aware of any extra support I may require, trips to the doctor or other health-related appointments which may pop up during work hours and generally just try to maintain an open line of communication.

For some thyroid patients, it may help to consider their job and if it's really suitable given their health situation. For example, are the hours ideal? I found that shift work never sat well with me, when my body runs so much better on routine. I've come to recognise that my perfect number of working hours match a part time role. It wasn't an easy decision to come down from full time work to part time, but I did it gradually, until I reached the point that I saw a good balance. This change in hours allowed me to have a much better work-life balance as I was no longer spending all my time at home sleeping until I went back to work the next morning, however, we did have to replan our finances and work out how we could afford to do this. You may find it helps to discuss these kinds of ideas with the thyroid patient in *your* life. Not everyone can afford to decrease their hours at work, so as a loved one, you should be included in this discussion early on so you can work out the right balance together.

Flexible working may also be worth considering, asking whether the employer is happy for them to move their working hours around to compensate for doctor's appointments or blood tests, will provide everyone with a more beneficial working arrangement.

Work from home jobs are something that I've also considered in the past, as I've been in offices that are too cold, drafty and noisy, which, when having thyroid and adrenal issues, were really hard to work in as I couldn't concentrate and perform at my optimal best. Remote working can be great if there are mobility concerns with their hypothyroidism or their condition is just better managed in a familiar environment.

You can also help the thyroid patient in your life consider the type of work they do, keeping in mind what they enjoy doing and find fulfilling.

Working can be more difficult for those with hypothyroidism and there's no shame in them adjusting their work situation so that it allows a better quality of life and with this, they'll be able to have more time and energy to do more of what they love with you.

However, if your loved one ever feels discriminated at work, based on their health condition/s, they have a right to complain and you should support them in this.

In the UK, if someone thinks they've been unfairly discriminated against, then they should try to raise it with the person, line manager, or even talk to Acas or Citizens Advice, or a trade union representative, if things cannot be sorted out informally. You might be able to take a claim to an employment tribunal for discrimination.

Check if they can get legal aid to help with legal costs. Employers must follow the law on preventing discrimination at work. If you're in another country, you can find information on discrimination at work online, but sadly we can't cover all countries in this little book! Just know that it isn't OK for someone to be treated unfairly and that they do have rights.

Adam's Insights

I witnessed Rachel forcing herself to get ready and go to work on days when she really should have been at home taking care of her health. She's hugely determined to be 'like everyone else' and carry on, but at times this only compounded the problem. Not wanting to let others down, she drove her health into a worse state.

On days when I would drop her off at work on the way to my workplace, I would watch her leave the car and wonder how on Earth she'd got herself there when I could see how unwell she was. If I was half as unwell as she was I would have called in sick. And I think that's part of the problem. Just because they live with a chronic health condition every day, it doesn't dilute how huge the effects can be.

Some mornings, I thought to myself, 'I wouldn't trust her to make me a cup of tea in this state' as I watched her struggle to get herself ready for work, yet she'd go into the office to write reports, do data inputting and other tasks that required her to be on top form for accuracy.

In the beginning, I didn't really get it. I did encourage her to go to work when I should have encouraged her to stay at home. Before I understood the true extent of thyroid disease, I couldn't grasp how she said she felt so unwell so often. But I learnt to trust her judgement and even sometimes be the one to tell her to take today off and try again tomorrow.

A Day at Home Sick

If your loved one with hypothyroidism has to take a day off work due to their health condition, then please know that avoiding judgement and instead asking if you can help will be a lot more productive.

Most sick days with hypothyroidism and/or Hashimoto's tend to be due to flare ups (which we covered in Chapter 4). Heavy fatigue and flu-type symptoms are commonly reported and can impact the ability to not only work, but even physically get to work or get out of bed. Days like this should be treated as seriously as other illnesses such as the flu and implications that it 'can't be that bad' are harmful.

I never like taking time off work due to my thyroid condition. It makes me feel rubbish. It makes me feel like a failure and I beat myself up about it. It's also not always easy to predict when a flare up will occur and I may literally only know on the morning of work.

Encouraging us to take care of ourselves by following the information on flares in Chapter 4 will go a long way to helping us recover more smoothly and get back to work sooner. Of course, thyroid conditions *can* be managed and controlled so that they needn't affect quality of life hugely, but it may well take the thyroid patient in your life quite a bit of time to get to that point and even when they do, flare ups can still occur.

Part Four: Support for Those Supporting Others

Support for the loved ones of those with hypothyroidism.

Chapter 18: Looking After Your Own Mental Health

"Taking care of yourself means keeping your own cup full. If you don't have a full cup, you have nothing left to give or share with others." - Adam Gask

By Adam

Unless you have the ability to manage your own mental health and well-being when trying to support someone with a chronic illness, it can put an incredible strain on you and your relationship.

As is the aim of this very book, we want your relationship to thrive - whether it's romantic, friendship, familial or another form of relationship - but the foundation of this must contain support for you too.

While supporting someone whose physical, and often mental health is struggling, you will also need to be mindful of your own mental health and well-being.

Resources that can prove useful include books and websites (such as those listed at the end of this book) as well as online communities and forums (such as the 'Loved Ones Of Those With Hypothyroidism' Facebook Group). There are groups for people supporting loved ones with health conditions both online and in person. A quick internet search will connect you with them. It can be really helpful to connect with other people in a similar situation to you. I can't stress enough, that knowing you are not alone in all of this, really *can* help.

It can also be useful to speak openly to friends and family about your experiences as someone who supports a chronically ill person. This is probably best done by confiding in no more than a couple of reliable people with whom you can trust to listen without judgement and not repeat your conversations. The last thing you want is for the person with hypothyroidism in your life to think that you're talking about them negatively behind their back and for people to gossip. Choose wisely and make sure you can trust them to be discreet.

I also found that at times I had to learn to help Rachel outside of being her partner. Essentially, looking at the situation and *her* situation without focusing on the fact that the woman I deeply care for is in pain. And that's hard. Getting myself upset about Rachel being upset, wasn't going to solve anything, but instead likely just make things worse. I'm not suggesting bottling up your feelings, but as someone who has been there, I can assure you this isn't healthy either. Reminding myself to stay grounded and focused on the task at hand, which was to get her back on to the road of recovery, was far more productive.

What helped my mental health through all of this was a lot of well-known techniques. Learning about mindfulness, giving yoga and meditation a go (don't knock it until you try it), and other exercise. I have a phrase that I use a lot, both with Rachel and others. I call it 'Taking Your Brain Out'. This is where you do an activity to quieten the mind and 'Take it out' by doing something else. This could be reading, playing a game, going for a run, literally anything which allows the mind to shift focus, even just for a small amount of time.

There may be times when you feel lost, lonely, frustrated, confused and angry at the current situation. It's actually important to not brush these feelings aside or under the carpet, but instead acknowledge them and be mindful of them. It's OK to not be OK, too. Acknowledge the feeling and then let it pass in a healthy way. It can also be worthwhile to discuss your feelings with your loved one. At the end of the day, the mental health of both people is important. This can feel hard, almost like you are adding an extra burden. But in my experience the loved one knows you are not superhuman, they know you are flesh and bone like them, so opening up and admitting your struggles can make them feel, in a strange way, relatable.

If you feel as if you would benefit from the support of a therapist or counsellor, please do reach out to these people and know that it isn't 'wrong' to need support in the form of counselling, therapy or even medication for mental health. Both Rachel and I feel that the stigma around these topics needs to be banished.

Make time for yourself and ensure that you maintain key parts of your own identity. As well as someone caring for another, you may also play 5-aside football, enjoy reading, building computers, gardening etc. Retain your own individuality, but be honest - I know people who would use this as an excuse to not face and address issues, too. It's all about balance.

It is also important to shift your mindset to a more fluid outlook. If you approach the situation thinking that the thyroid patient in your life need only tick ten things off a checklist and they'll be all 'fixed', you're setting yourself up to fail. This journey together is going to need ongoing maintenance and commitment, which can feel scary at times, but, as with all things, you do get better at navigating the choppy waters of supporting others.

Further Mental Health Support:

UK

Mind
Phone: 0300 123 3393
Website: https://www.mind.org.uk/

Samaritans
Phone: 116 123
Website: https://www.samaritans.org/

CALM
Phone: 0800 58 58 58
Website: https://www.thecalmzone.net/

Young Minds
Text: YM to 85258
Website: https://youngminds.org.uk/

US

Lines for Life
Phone: 800-273-8255
Website: https://www.linesforlife.org/

National Suicide Prevention Lifeline
Phone: 1800 273 TALK (8255)
Website: https://www.suicidepreventionlifeline.org/

We unfortunately can't list helplines for all countries, but please know that you can find your local support services with a quick internet search. Please reach out for support if you need to.

Epilogue

18th May 2019, Bruges, Belgium

By Adam

I write this final note, by the waterside of Minnewater Lake, Bruges, on our first wedding anniversary. We have spent this trip cycling, walking and laughing.

The journey Rachel and I have been on since her initial thyroid diagnosis has been far more of a rollercoaster than I ever could have imagined. Her hypothyroidism has changed our relationship for better and for worse over the years. The difference from where we were a few years ago, knowing nothing about this disease and all the struggles that come with it, to where we are today, cannot be understated. We are no longer the people we were back then, but not in a bad way.

Living and being with someone who is hypothyroid is not easy, and certainly not your 'normal' loving/support role. It takes far more effort than anyone would like to admit publicly, but one that should be discussed. However, with the things discussed in this book and Rachel's other work and resources, we both hope that your relationship, whatever that may be, can flourish and that your loved one is able to get their thyroid disease under control one day too. There have been plenty of times in the last four years where I myself didn't believe that would be possible, as I've seen and experienced how hard this can be for everyone involved.

Today feels like an appropriate day to write this epilogue to our book, as today, Rachel tamed her hypothyroidism.

Many years ago, Rachel wasn't able to do the simplest of tasks due to her thyroid condition, and my overriding memory of this is one of when she once fell down the stairs and I had to carry her back up to bed. I knew something was very wrong and it was the night we decided to take responsibility for getting her health back on track. She has hated all forms of stairs ever since, but today, she scaled the Belfry Tower of Bruges (nearly 400 steps) and made it with a smile on her face. A feat I never truly believed I would ever see her complete.

Today, *she's* the one in control of her health, and her thyroid isn't controlling *her* anymore. This is where I want all loved ones to be with the hypothyroid one in their lives. I want everyone to tame this disease and return to a sense of 'normality', whatever that means to you. I hope that this book helps you both on this journey and I hope it reassures you that it can be done. We *can* have strengthened relationships and help our loved ones back to good health. The version of myself a few years ago wouldn't have believed we'd be travelling the world and getting up to so many adventures with the way Rachel's health once was.

But yet here we are. Your loved one *and* your relationship with them can thrive despite the third wheel of thyroid disease.

I wish you both every success.

Best,

Adam

Sources of Further Information and Support

"Knowledge is power." - Sir Francis Bacon

As well as Rachel's website and supporting social media platforms (Facebook, Instagram, Twitter) the below can be utilised to gain more knowledge in to hypothyroidism and Hashimoto's.

Those mentioned below are not necessarily endorsed by us and we cannot control the content or opinions expressed on external websites. They are listed for you and your loved one to explore.

Please also consider leaving an online review of **this** book, *You, Me and Hypothyroidism*, so that other people can gauge if it will help them in their own journey. Amazon and Goodreads are popular places to do this.

Websites

In alphabetical order:

Dr Nikolas Hedberg

Dr Hedberg is a well-respected and praised functional medicine practitioner. With lots of great articles and podcasts on his website, there is plenty of information to digest.

Holtorf Medical Group

The HMG specialises in optimising quality of life and being

medical detectives to uncover the underlying cause of symptoms. Their website showcases this level of knowledge with scientifically backed up articles which are shared often across social media.

Hypothyroid Mom

Dana at Hypothyroid Mom went through the traumatic experience of losing her unborn child when doctors failed to monitor her hypothyroidism correctly. She started blogging and advocating in pursuit of changing thyroid treatment and saving lives. She often features doctors as content providers to her blog.

Mary Shomon: Thyroid Patient Advocate

Mary Shomon has a very popular Facebook page and writes for various websites. Once hyperthyroid who is now hypothyroid, she advocates for both.

Stop The Thyroid Madness

STTM focus mainly on the power of NDT medication in the treatment of hypothyroidism and is largely built on patient experiences, encouraging thyroid patients to share their stories and learn from one another.

The Butterfly Effect Blog

The Butterfly Effect Blog is a health and wellness website dedicated to providing research and patient-to-patient advice on healing and dealing with chronic illness. It is created by Victoria, who has Hashimoto's.

The National Academy of Hypothyroidism

The NAH is a non-profit, multidisciplinary medical society dedicated to the dissemination of new information on the diagnosis and treatment of hypothyroidism, mainly in the USA. It is run by a group of thyroidologists, headed by Kent Holtorf M.D., David Brownstein, M.D., Denis Wilson, M.D., Michael Freidman, N.D., and Mary Shomon.

Articles and blogs on all things thyroid are written in a format that is easy to understand and digest.

Thoughtful Thyroid

Thoughtful Thyroid was created by Rachel Hill of The Invisible Hypothyroidism and Nadha Hassen from Thyroid Transitions, who have come together to bring a thoughtful, mindful approach to healing from thyroid disease by empowering fellow thyroid patients and their loved ones via online courses that enable learning, understanding, good health and wellness.

ThyroidChange

ThyroidChange is an organisation that seeks to improve the diagnosis and treatment of thyroid conditions. They are a grass-roots movement for better thyroid care. Thyroid Change have a website full of useful articles written by doctors and thyroid advocates.

Thyroid Nation

Thyroid Nation focuses on uplifting readers with positive articles and stories that present information learnt from personal experiences. A lot of the articles are also based around lifestyle changes and factors that can greatly improve thyroid health.

Thyroid Patient Advocacy

A UK charity, TPA is an independent organisation that also works towards establishing better diagnosis and treatment of hypothyroidism in patients. Dr Barry Durrant-Peatfield is a Trustee and Dr Kent Holtorf a Medical Adviser. There are countless hugely informative articles written by various doctors and healthcare professionals on the site, with information for both patients and doctors.

Thyroid Pharmacist, Izabella Wentz

Izabella Wentz is a well-respected pharmacist who also developed Hashimoto's. Through her own determination and knowledge as a medical professional, she has managed to reverse her autoimmune condition by implementing lifestyle and diet changes that she shares in her book and on her website.

Thyroid Refresh

Thyroid Refresh is an online platform that makes living a thyroid healthy lifestyle into a game. Thyroid30 is a 30-day wellness adventure that focuses on living a healthier thyroid lifestyle.

Thyroid UK

Thyroid UK are a Thyroid Charity in the United Kingdom. They work on improving the diagnosis and treatment of thyroid disease and are often at the front of campaigns and research drives.

Books

We recognise that investing in a lot of books can be expensive, so it's also worth knowing that Rachel has reviewed all of these and more, on her website at TheInvisibleHypothyroidism.com/category/book-reviews/ so you can get a good idea of whether certain books would be beneficial to you or your loved one, before spending your hard-earned cash.

In alphabetical order:

Adrenal Fatigue: The 21st Century Stress Syndrome by James L. Wilson, N.D, D.C, Ph.D

Beyond The Pill by Dr Jolene Brighten

Be Your Own Thyroid Advocate: When You're Sick and Tired of Being Sick and Tired by Rachel Hill AKA The Invisible Hypothyroidism

Diagnosis and Management of Hypothyroidism by Gordon R B Skinner, MD, DSc, FRCPath, FRCOG
Hashimoto's Thyroiditis: Lifestyle Interventions for Finding and Treating the Root Cause by Izabella Wentz PharmD

Stop The Thyroid Madness: A Patient Revolution Against Decades of Inferior Thyroid Treatment by Janie A. Bowthorpe, M.Ed

The 30-Minute Thyroid Cookbook: 125 Healing Recipes for Hypothyroidism and Hashimoto's by Emily Kyle MS, RDN, CDN, CLT and Rachel Hill AKA The Invisible Hypothyroidism

The End of Chronic Fatigue by Zana Carver Ph.D and Gina Heath INHC

The Hormone Cure by Sara Gottfried, MD

What You Must Know About Hashimoto's Disease by Brittany Henderson, MD, ECNU, and Allison Futterman

Why Do I STILL Have Thyroid Symptoms? When My Lab Tests Are Normal.. by Datis Kharrazian, DHSc, DC, MS

Your Healthy Pregnancy with Thyroid Disease by Dana Trentini and Mary Shomon

Your Thyroid and how to keep it healthy.. The Great Thyroid Scandal and How to Survive it by Dr Barry Durrant-Peatfield

RACHEL HILL & ADAM GASK

Appendix

[1] Amino, N. 1988, *Autoimmunity and hypothyroidism*, viewed 12th July 2019,
<https://www.ncbi.nlm.nih.gov/pubmed/3066320>

[2] *National Academy of Clinical Biochemistry 2002, Laboratory Medicine Practice Guidelines: Laboratory Support for the Diagnosis and Monitoring of Thyroid Disease,* viewed 5th June 2019
<http://www.aacc.org/sitecollectiondocuments/nacb/lmpg/thyroid/thyroid-fullversion.pdf>

[3] Hollowell, J.G., Staehling, N.W., Flanders, W.D., Hannon, W.H., Gunter, E.W., Spencer, C.A., Braverman, L.E. 2002, *Serum TSH, T4, and thyroid antibodies in the United States population (1988 to 1994): National Health and Nutrition Examination Survey (NHANES III),* viewed 5th June 2019
<https://www.ncbi.nlm.nih.gov/pubmed/11836274>

[4] *Guidance - Prescribing of Liothyronine (RMOC),* viewed 5th June 2019
<https://www.sps.nhs.uk/wp-content/uploads/2018/11/RMOC-Liothyronine-Guidance-v2.0-final-1.pdf>

[5] Larisch, Midgley JEM, Dietrich JW, Hoermann R., 2018,*Symptomatic Relief is Related to Serum Free Triiodothyronine Concentrations during Follow-up in Levothyroxine-Treated Patients with Differentiated Thyroid Cancer,* viewed 5th June 2019
<https://www.ncbi.nlm.nih.gov/pubmed/29396968>

[6] Viewed 12th July 2019 <https://www.btf-thyroid.org/information/leaflets/42-congenital-hypothyroidism-guide>

[7] Viewed 4th July 2019
<https://thyroidpharmacist.com/articles/pregnancy-announcement/>

[8] Viewed 4th July 2019
<https://butyoudontlooksick.com/articles/written-by-christine/the-spoon-theory/>

[9] Schuder S.E, 2005, *Stress-induced hypocortisolemia diagnosed as psychiatric disorders responsive to hydrocortisone replacement,* viewed 4th July 2019 <//www.ncbi.nlm.nih.gov/pubmed/16399913>

[10]Abalovich M, Amino N, Barbour LA, Cobin RH, De Groot LJ, Glinoer D, Mandel SJ, Stagnaro-Green A, 2007, *Management of Thyroid Dysfunction During Pregnancy and Postpartum: An Endocrine Society Clinical Practice Guideline.* Viewed 4th July 2019 <https://www.ncbi.nlm.nih.gov/pubmed/17948378>

[11] Viewed 19th July 2019
<https://www.nahypothyroidism.org/newborns-and-congenital-hypothyroidism/>

[12] Viewed 19th July 2019 <https://www.btf-thyroid.org/information/leaflets/42-congenital-hypothyroidism-guide>

[13] Viewed 12th July 2019
<https://www.theinvisiblehypothyroidism.com/how-i-got-my-hashimotos-in-to-remission/>